A Systemic Approach to Integrative Counselling

This book presents systemic psychotherapy to integrative counsellors by using the most common counselling modalities and turning them into systemic approaches.

A Systemic Approach to Integrative Counselling teaches systemic theory and techniques gradually, delving into various ways for integrative counsellors to think from a systemic perspective, reframing a client's presenting problem as emerging from relationships and social context. The chapters discuss how to combine person-centred counselling with a systemic outlook, how to combine psychodynamic theory with ideas about circularity and relationships, and outlines ways to use cognitive-behavioural therapy, action techniques, drama techniques, gestalt therapy, and many counselling approaches systemically with individual clients. The author's conversational writing, accompanied with case studies and in-depth explanations of counselling techniques and theories, makes the material interactive and accessible.

A Systemic Approach to Integrative Counselling will provide qualified and trainee counsellors with an in-depth systemic outlook on counselling modalities. It is also a helpful guide for scholars and researchers in related fields.

Rick Murphy is a Systemic Psychotherapist and Senior Lecturer in Psychology at the University of Northampton, UK.

A Systemic Approach to Integrative Counselling

Rick Murphy

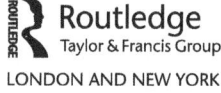

Routledge
Taylor & Francis Group

LONDON AND NEW YORK

Designed cover image: Getty Images via kubkoo

First published 2025
by Routledge
4 Park Square, Milton Park, Abingdon, Oxon OX14 4RN

and by Routledge
605 Third Avenue, New York, NY 10158

Routledge is an imprint of the Taylor & Francis Group, an informa business

British Library Cataloguing-in-Publication Data
A catalogue record for this book is available from the British Library

ISBN: 9781032770048 (hbk)
ISBN: 9781032770024 (pbk)
ISBN: 9781003480808 (ebk)

DOI: 10.4324/9781003480808

Typeset in Times New Roman
by Deanta Global Publishing Services, Chennai, India

Contents

Introduction

Counselling is a moral and virtuous profession that tries to end the psychological suffering of people who find themselves stuck in hopeless and distressing realities. There are many thoughtful ideas about how to put a stop to the worry, the depression, and the sense of despair felt by our clients, all of whom hope that by speaking and being with us in therapy they will become freer and happier in the outside world. The sense of importance this responsibility places on our skills and therapeutic interventions can pressure us into using a narrow way of working, being anchored to certain specialisms, theories, and techniques. I hope this book will bring out some of the playfulness and creativity needed to give counsellors and trainees the permission to use the responsibility we have for our clients' wellbeing to create inventive and meaningful practices.

A new perspective on counselling has been growing since the late 1980s. Many therapists moved away from individual concepts like personality and self-growth towards the perspective that counselling issues are symptoms of human systems, of relationships. Systemic concepts remain relatively untapped resources for integrative counsellors, and this book presents a model for combining counselling and systemic modalities into an integrative framework. I am calling this model Systemic Integrative Counselling and in this chapter I describe the theoretical roots of the model.

Using systemic psychotherapy as a foundation for counselling is made possible by a little-known theory that profoundly questions the assumption that counselling and systemic models have strict boundaries. It merges, borrows, and integrates counselling techniques from one model and another. And, as much as being an exciting and enriching tool for the counsellor, it creates counselling techniques that are truly integrative. The model is called "AMT", which stands for Approach, Method, and Technique. The theory was developed in the early 1990s by John Burnham, a family therapist and systemic author who wanted to deconstruct counselling and psychotherapy models into their basic parts. Three ingredients of a counselling model emerged, and these were the Approach or set of guiding principles and theories; the Method or way of working within an organisation or counselling context; and the Techniques or set of skills and interventions. Who would

DOI: 10.4324/9781003480808-1

have thought that such a simple framework could be the key to unifying systemic and counselling modalities?

Let's take an example counselling model to deconstruct using the AMT approach, such as a model that centres on the client's experience. The top level, the "approach", is linked with guiding principles like humanism, which is the theory that people have innate capacities for self-growth. In such a client- or person-centred model, the middle level, the "method", is one of individual counselling, providing a stable and private weekly space. The counselling routine allows the therapist to become a relationship for self-growth. The lower level, the "techniques", within this method are things like open questions, paraphrasing and summarising the client's words. These three techniques fit neatly into the methods and approach of a person-centred counselling approach because they match the guiding principles of humanism, trusting the client to grow organically with the process (Table 0.1).

AMT separates the person-centred modality into its component parts, like breaking down a Lego house into different blocks. The AMT model can deconstruct all counselling modalities and integrate them into new models. For instance, with cognitive-behavioural therapy (CBT), AMT might take the roof of the CBT house to be the theory that mental health is the outcome of habituated cognitive-behavioural cycles and theorise that behaviour modification and psychoeducation instigate change. The body of the house, or the methods in this model, would slightly differ from the person-centred house, being manualised and time-limited rather than non-directive and open-ended. And the base of the house, the techniques, are based on psychoeducation worksheets, challenging intrusive thinking, and using homework tasks and role-plays (Table 0.2).

Table 0.1 Person-Centred Therapy

Approach	Humanism: the client has the capacity for growth. The client's experience should be centred on and guide the counsellor
Method	Weekly non-directed 50-minute sessions in a counselling room with client and counsellor. Open-ended
Technique	Open questions Paraphrasing Summarising

Table 0.2 Cognitive Behavioural Therapy

Approach	Cognitive theory: thinking affects feelings and behaviours Psychoeducation: insight into cognitive behavioural cycles and negative thinking or behaviour patterns instigates change
Method	Weekly manualised 50-minute session in a counselling room with client and counsellor. Time-limited
Technique	Cognitive behavioural worksheet Role-play Thought diary Homework tasks

Table 0.3 Client-Centred Behavioural Therapy

Approach	Cognitive theory: thinking affects feelings and behaviours
	Psychoeducation: insight into cognitive behavioural cycles and negative thinking or behaviour patterns instigates change
Method	Weekly manualised 50-minute session in a counselling room with client and counsellor. Time-limited
Technique	Open questions
	Paraphrasing
	Cognitive-behavioural worksheet
	Role-play
	Thought diary

AMT thus separates counselling modalities into approaches, methods, and techniques, but is more than a load of blocks hierarchically arranged into counselling modalities. As with a Lego structure, it enables counsellors to move something from one model to another and create new structures. And this is the revolution of thought that is needed for a systemic approach to integrative counselling. In a situation where the cognitive-behavioural style becomes stuck when working with a client, the counsellor can borrow techniques from person-centred counselling and try a new, integrative approach, borrowing techniques but staying within a cognitive theory. We might coin a new therapeutic school and call the approach something like "client-centred behavioural therapy" (Table 0.3).

If you look carefully, Table 0.3 highlights an important perspective. AMT addresses the position that counselling modalities have become straightjacketed and stereotyped into, which is the perceived incompatibility of different counselling modalities. CBT gets called sterile. Person-centred gets called wishy washy and impractical. Psychodynamic gets called bossy and judgemental. Systemic gets called resource-heavy and emotionally detached. When probing into the experiences of trainees, colleagues, and clients—the people who make such claims— often the problem is with the rigidity with which the counsellor (or trainer!) held on to the techniques and theories. Having the freedom to move between modalities releases counsellors and clients from entrenched problems.

The counsellor needn't drop their guiding theory and way of working. They need only adopt techniques from another theoretical household. For instance, a CBT counsellor can remain within a cognitive framework but use more open questions and paraphrasing in their approach. Taking five minutes to show unconditional positive regard towards a client's experience, to use empathy to increase the client's awareness of their thoughts and feelings, can be a way of unpacking cognitive-behavioural cycles. No need to mention humanism and self-actualisation. And this would certainly undermine the detachment that some clients experience with manualised cognitive therapies.

Equally, the person-centred therapist can imagine the structure of a cognitive-behavioural worksheet while they work with a client. When the window of opportunity opens, asking the client open questions about how their thinking is affecting

Table 0.4 Client-Centred CBT

Approach	Humanism: the client has the capacity for growth
	Non-directiveness: the client's experience should be centred on and guide the counsellor
Method	Weekly non-directed 50-minute sessions in a counselling room with client and counsellor. Open-ended
Technique	Cognitive-behavioural orientation when client leads in this direction
	Open questions
	Paraphrasing

their feelings-in-the-moment is completely consistent with client-centred practice. It does not need a directive worksheet, just a practical orientation of the therapist to assist the client in becoming aware of their cognitive-behavioural cycles when the client leads them in the direction of thoughts or feelings. No need to steer the session and psychoeducate (Table 0.4).

The AMT model highlights a way forward in combining different modalities into new uncharted approaches. Much of what is labelled as integrative is in fact eclectic or pluralist. That is, there are many counselling approaches separated by a theoretical and technical gulf. I, for example, am a systemic psychotherapist and I trained for four years without a concept of empathy in my university reading. This astonishes my counselling students!

It is a shame that the reverse is also true, that systemic thinking has not yet been integrated into the counselling field, because it has the potential to enrich counselling practice. In the way that I have used AMT to integrate from a person-centred modality to a CBT modality, I have written this book as a dialogue between systemic and counselling ideas, taking the reader on a journey through the full catalogue of systemic concepts and techniques, integrating them into the most widespread counselling modalities. This is not a talk on the merits of one counselling approach, but an alternative view of counselling that turns its back on the point of view of separation and boundaries towards the view of connections.

I will assume the reader has no knowledge of counselling or systemic ideas. Assuming no prior knowledge will help present counselling models clearly and sharpen understanding of familiar and unfamiliar ways of thinking. By the end of the book, counsellors will have new ways of seeing their favoured models and new ways of using their favoured models within a systemic framework. Systemic readers may reframe and rethink many of their systemic ideas through the lens of counselling modalities and as such gain new insights and techniques for their therapy practice. I am careful not to categorise systemic and counselling models as better or worse, simply to guide the reader through the different approaches and techniques while comparing them to establish multiple ways of working, and, in a word, to "integrate" counselling and systemic models into a single unified approach. The final chapter will introduce this under the title: Systemic Integrative Counselling, or SIC for short. But before we arrive at that conclusion, we will outline the basics of systems theory and sketch a pathway for how to combine these exciting and mutually reinforcing counselling modalities.

Further reading

Burnham, J. (1999). Approach, method, technique: Making distinctions and creating connections from human systems. *The Journal of Systemic Consultation and Management, 3*(1), 3–26.

Faris, A., & Ooijen, E. Van (2012). *Integrative counselling and psychotherapy: A textbook.* London: Routledge.

Lapworth, P., & Sills, C. (2009). *Integration in counselling & psychotherapy: Developing a personal approach.* London: Sage.

Russell, W., Breunlin, D., & Sahebi, B. (2022). *Integrative systemic therapy.* London: Routledge.

Chapter 1

Systems Theory

The world falsely appears to us as a collection of separated objects. In truth, the shape, size, character, scent, strength, weakness, beauty, and temperature of an object or life form is deeply connected with a rich history of development within a system. An ecosystem. A social system. A solar system. A living system. Everything is interwoven inside a web of relationships and connections. In this chapter we explain the ideas that inspired people to think about systems and we take a tour through the winding history of modern systems theory.

The term "systems theory" was not in circulation until 1893. Emile Durkheim, a doctorate student, attempted to answer the fascinating question, why do societies rise and fall over time? He worked out that human societies are more like ants than polar bears; instead of a solitary lifestyle, humans are social animals that thrive on giving each person a role to play. Explaining why somebody becomes anti-social, say, a criminal or psychotic, was hitherto explained by demonic forces and broken souls. The new systems theory found that when a person is not integrated properly into the social system, the fact of having no meaningful role pushes them to the brink of crime and mental illness. In fact, crime and mental illness become their role.

A person's behaviour, mental life, and society were suddenly linked. Sociology was discovered as a science for examining how human identity is created from social forces. One of the first people to take on the name of sociologist was Talcott Parsons. He developed a theory beyond Durkheim's in which social roles, and not the specific people in those roles, kept the structure of society solid. This put forward a radical view, that important people like the friendly neighbourhood doctor are not only nice and caring people who seek to keep others healthy. A doctor's internal motivation, their sense of their own morality, is formed out of a social role that keeps people healthy for them to fulfil other important social roles. Maintaining the social structure was shown to be vital for a thriving society and people were shown to act in the interests of the society, and unconsciously. This structural functionalism, which is the name given to this process by Parsons, explained that independence is an illusion and that people's skills, personalities, and even their mental ill-health serve social functions.

DOI: 10.4324/9781003480808-2

Parsons found that social life is kept stable by attaining goals, maintaining social patterns, adapting to change, and integrating people into the system. If any of these four pillars of the system broke down, the society crumbled. The work of Ludwig von Bertalanffy pulled systems theory away from human systems to model how systems work in their own right. He termed this "general systems theory", or GST, and defined a system as a group of things that work together in a complex network or whole. Although very abstract, this gave Bertalanffy licence to name and describe a variety of systems. There are human systems, ecosystems, family systems, mathematical systems, respiratory systems, legal systems, living systems, political systems. All such networks of interacting components were describable in terms of some straightforward concepts. This immediately pushed sociology into a subsystem of general systems theory.

How does society remain stable? Why do the social norms not collapse? What supplies society with its fuel to keep going? How does a system evolve and change?

Although the properties of a system were now known, it was not clear to us how systems change over time. Obviously on some level people move about and do things to alter their relationships but what influences behaviour change? The renowned systems theorist Donella Meadows invited us to think about the behaviour of systems using an example from nature, that of the deer population. In deer society, when a deer is born, the population of deer goes up. The more births, the more deer. Thus, the size of the deer population is linked with annual births and deaths. So, the deer population is regulated by the number of deer born minus the number of deer that die each year. But what systemic factors influence births and deaths each year?

Some deer die by natural causes and some die by accidents. But importantly, the deer population is also hunted by calculating predators. The surrounding population of hungry wolves, bears, foxes, and mountain lions is interrelated to the deer population. Meadows showed that as the number of deer grows there is more food for the hungry predators and the abundance of deer meat increases the predator population. And here's the important thing: the deer population reaches a critical point at which it starts to decrease. Now the deer population, being eaten by the surrounding carnivores, shrinks to a point of almost being off the menu. And, with the decrease in the number of deer, the predator population substantially drops. The deer-predator populations have what's known in systems theory as circular causation. From an evolutionary perspective, the long legs of the deer and the sharp teeth of the lynx develop in tandem; as one gets more cunning the other gets fiercer. As one gets fiercer, the other gets more cunning. The individual property of being fierce or cunning is tied up in the predator-prey *system*. And so genetically and population-wise, the deer and the predator populations co-evolve within a closed system (see Figure 1.1).

But what does systems theory have to do with counselling?

The question above invites us to consider how the client's world presents itself to us as a series of things or events. A person treated them unkindly. They have an unshakeable anxiety problem. And this presentation of the problem obscures the

Deer population

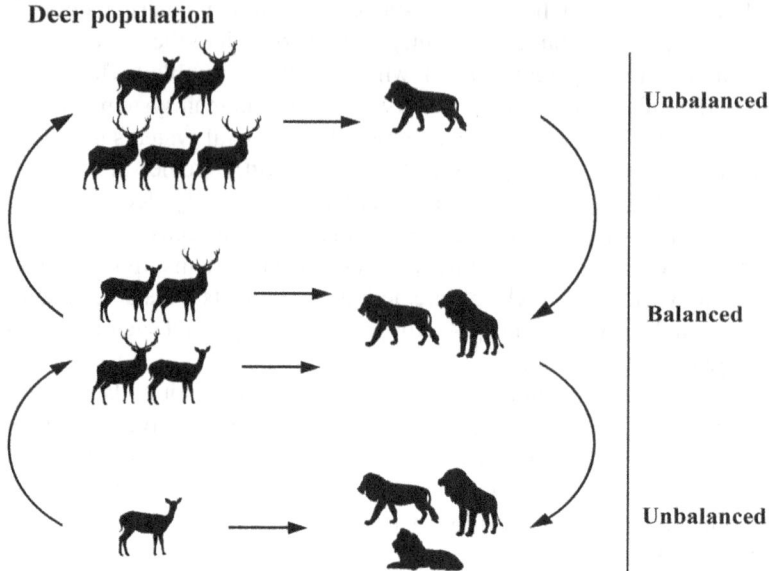

Figure 1.1 The Deer Population

system in which the events are part of. For instance, seeing a deer being eaten as an event gives us little predicative power over events that led to this situation and that will happen in the future. Seeing this as part of a system, however, opens up the possibility of looking behind and ahead, of predicting how the event is mapped out in a system. With counselling clients, and here's the connection, this is also true of the event of anxiety, anger, suicidality, and depression. As one person in, say, an intimate relationship becomes closer and more dependent, the other person becomes more distant and independent, with wellbeing levels and dependency levels keeping the relationship stable and balanced even when psychological experience suffers. Systemic theorists such as Murray Bowen and Gregory Bateson have found the same circularity, the same systemic loops, when looking at mental health problems. Human anxiety is like a deer's flight-response from a predator, it says something about the systemic situation for the client.

Out of this work sprung system dynamics theory, which clarified the different structures of a system. First, a system must be named and described as a whole. For instance, the predator-prey system. The political system. The sibling system. Or the couple system. Then the individual components of that system are described, such as the psychological characteristics of brothers and sisters, the hunting patterns of lynxes and lions, and the closeness of a couple. Then the feedback loops are examined, which are closed chains of causation. For example, the more a person asks for closeness, the more the other demands distance, which causally generates arguments. The arguments are a form of feedback to the members of the couple about the state of their couple system. After more arguments, the members of the couple negotiate the correct level of closeness that is emotionally safe for everyone. Some couples are strengthened by the feedback loop, and some couples crumble under the pressure. This artificial selection of closeness is like natural selection in that systems that survive are those things which function well to balance the competing demands of its members. Over time, a balance will be struck between different elements of the system, whereby the system will run through predictable cycles, like with the deer-predator population, or settle on some happy medium between the components, such as having more understanding and responsiveness towards a need for privacy and a need for proximity in a sexual relationship. A feedback loop is the basic mechanism of a system and maintains the system's stability. The stability of the system is called its equilibrium or its homeostasis. In this example, the wellbeing of each partner is regulated by matching individual factors with factors to do with their position in the cycle of negotiating closeness and distance. For instance, in the early relationship, we know if one is anxious then the other is probably withdrawn. The counselling issue, seen from the perspective of systems theory, is the issue of how a relationship pattern creates mental unrest.

The psychologist Urie Bronfenbrenner applied systems theory to psychological systems. Exchanging the deer model for the child development model, he saw that when a child is born, their psychological systems shape who they become. At first the child is already an organised system. The body is made from a skeletal system, muscular system, nervous system, respiratory system, and digestive system. The child must keep their blood temperature constant in the changing climate of their environment. And a reminder that the stability of the system is called its homeostasis, with people tending to achieve temperature homeostasis, which means preserving the same temperature in the body, around 37 degrees Celsius, using feedback loops from the temperature outside the body. Thus, the person must sweat or shiver depending on the weather conditions.

Sweating and shivering are easy to understand as being symptoms of a systemic dynamic, perhaps because we are used to thinking about temperature in this way. The systemic view takes this simple case and applies it to all thoughts, behaviours, feelings, and characteristics of the client. This works because the child's organismic or biological system interacts with their higher-level social systems. First the child is born into a family. The tastes and textures they come to accept and reject in their digestive system are determined by the types of foods and cooking methods of the family. A family helps the child make sense of what it means to eat and the kinds of eating habits that are common. Do we eat cooked foods? Spicy foods? Takeaways? Meat? Do we sit at tables? Do we sit together routinely? The child habituates to the family environment, and the family, using feedback loops between members, maintains its homeostasis—keeping the roles of mother, father, son, daughter, and so on, in relative stability around eating behaviours and family life.

Similarly to the digestive system, the same is true of meaning and emotional systems. How do people respond to sadness in my family? Is anger acceptable?

Who responds to me when I need help? Is it always my mum? And why? The child interacts with their parents and their parents respond. Through this mutual responsive relationship process, an attachment system is developed in the child, serving as a template for their future intimate and social relationships.

Bronfenbrenner noticed that the systemic influence on the child's development did not stop there. It was obvious that the family is not really a closed system. The family values, the conversations about schooling, the engagement with peers, are all components of family life. System dynamics theory calls this an operationally closed system because the family, albeit it a network of people by itself, is influenced by being part of a community system. The family operates as a closed system but is part of a community of families. If the child looks outside the front door and see cars set on fire or green rolling landscapes, the type of parenting that is appropriate in the family system changes. Having a secure attachment is dysfunctional in a hostile group. Having an insecure attachment is dysfunctional in a loving group.

Communication between the family and the community regulates the kinds of values and expectations within the family (it keeps stability). Although the parents are the ones hugging, rejecting, or telling the child to eat healthily or say no to drugs, it is the community in which the family establishes the importance of one value in relation to another. The community creates a feedback loop with the family whereby social norms are expected and imposed. If social norms are unmet, neighbours will scorn, phone the police, and even try and have the family evicted or imprisoned. The child's bodily system is intimately tied up with their family system, and their family system is embedded within a community. Having worked out the puzzle of why people's individual characteristics vary with distinctive social patterns, such that people from one community and another tend to take on similar characteristics, some big questions remained; how does the community system develop? Where does its value system come from? How does the community keep hold of its balance?

The decision to live by a concrete high-rise estate or a detached mansion in the countryside is not simply a personal choice. Obviously! The society builds houses clumped together and spread apart according to factors like population size and budget. The national culture, if one of capitalism for example, will tend to create pockets of wealth and areas of poverty because these types of systems need a class of workers for labour and a class of rulers, politicians, bankers, and business executives. The society values capitalism or socialism, individualism or collectivism, for example, and these values sit dictatorially at the top of a social pyramid. In an individualistic society, where the ideal is for individual independence, there is more market for meals-for-one and people are likely to move away from their parents nearer the age of 18. The reverse is true if the society values togetherness and is sociocentric. Having a value system of independence in the United Kingdom means that by the age of 30 most people are expected to be married with children on the way, living in their own home. Economically, as we are finding out, this value system clashes with capitalism because landlords and governments make this financially unviable. Gentrification is a good example of this, where poorer areas are overtaken by middle-class people when suburban or desirable urban areas are financially out of their reach. This is a feedback loop and maintains the balance of social class. The poorer communities don't tend to benefit from the newer, snazzier shops. They tend to get priced out of their communities and remain poor. This too is social homeostasis, where although absolute poverty decreases over time, relative poverty between the rich and the poor remains stable. Each individual develops and adapts within complex environments.

How does systems theory link with counselling?

In the counselling clinic, the first conclusion from systems theory is that mental health is tied in with family and social expectations in the wider society. Meaning systems, in which culture shapes media, social expectations, feedback loops between spouses and friends, parents and children, are upheld by the society which evaluates the lower-down community and family systems according to its own values. There are feedback loops about attractiveness. Skills. The appropriate relationship status for your age. The definition of success and failure. Whether getting good grades is cool or nerdish. The pride of cleverness and the shame of stupidity. The right background for a high-paying job. The wrong background for fitting in socially. For an individual to experience a positive wellbeing they must play a role in their local social game where they are valued and validated for who they are. An individual is an experiencing and reacting being within a living-breathing social system. Bronfenbrenner calls his model the "ecological systems theory" or EST because it relates to how human identity and wellbeing are shaped within a hierarchical social arrangement. Feedback loops occur between the political and cultural dimensions, between the culture and the community, between the community and the family, and between the family and the individual. A person coming to counselling brings a layered social and systemic dilemma with them.

The result of viewing the system around the individual problem is to expand the client's understanding of their difficulties and create lives of heightened wellbeing and meaning. Peter Stratton, a systemic theorist and researcher, has reviewed the research and shown that the evidence base for reductions in problems like low mood and anxiety is extremely strong with a systemic approach, across an enormous variety of study designs and client issues. This is because the individual psychological experience is part of a circular world that creates social and psychological realities (see Figure 1.2). Nicholas Luhmann added a concept to systems theory called autopoiesis, which literally means self-creation. He noticed that human systems are structured by feedback loops that continually recreate themselves using the actions and states of mind of the individual people in the system. Thus, counselling clients are members of a social system in which their presenting problem both results from and contributes to creating social norms in society.

Over the past 80 years or so, this idea of circular causation, of social context to psychological problems, which is the principle of systems theory, has been translated into concepts to aid counsellors. The chapters that follow build on the work described here to demonstrate how systems theory integrates into the counselling

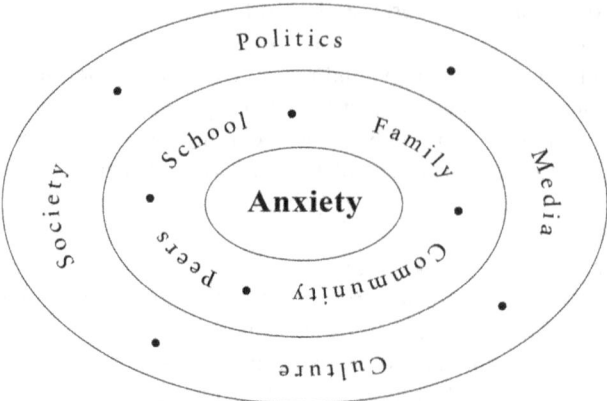

Figure 1.2 Anxiety in Society

field more generally. We will look at family systems, couple systems, friendship systems, communication systems, and social systems to show how the theories you have learned in this chapter help to generate practical tools for integrative counsellors.

Further Reading

Bertalanffy, L. von (1968). *General system theory: Foundation, development, application.* New York: George Braziller.

Bronfenbrenner, U. (1979). *The ecology of human development: Experiments by nature and design.* Cambridge, MA: Harvard University Press.

Carr, A., Pinquart, M., & Haun, M. W. (2020). Research-informed practice of systemic therapy. In M. Ochs, M. Borcsa, & J. Schweitzer (Eds.), *Systemic research in individual, couple and family therapy and Counseling.* Cham: Springer, pp. 319–347.

Durkheim, É. (1984). *The division of labour in society* (2nd ed.). New York: Macmillan.

Luhmann, N. (2013). *Introduction to systems theory.* Cambridge: Polity Press.

Meadows, D. (2009). *Thinking in systems.* Vermont: Chelsea Green Publishing.

Parsons, T. (1951). *The social system.* Glenco, IL: Free Press.

Stratton, P. (2016). *The evidence base of family therapy and systemic practice.* Warrington: Association of Family Therapy.

Chapter 2

System-Centred Counselling

Carl Rogers came up with a theory of personality. He predicted that, with the right ingredients, the individual person has a natural pull towards reaching their potential and appreciation for life. Happiness and contentment are dependent on feeling fulfilled and self-aware.

He was a humanistic psychologist who believed that people have free will and are self-determined, but only when their basic physical, psychological, and social needs are met. Any disturbances in needs for safety, social contact, and meaning in life would cause people to develop an inconsistent picture of themselves, holding obscure and contradictory inner beliefs that impair their experiences. It was natural for Carl Rogers to centre his approach on the whole person, in his famous person-centred or client-centred therapy, because helping the person to organise their experience, acknowledging their true thoughts and beliefs, makes them more likely to reach their potential and appreciation for life. In this chapter we describe Carl Rogers' person-centred theory and show you a way to integrate it with systems theory.

History tells us that, for Carl Rogers, the solution to the problem of disorganised experience and a diminished sense of self was to use three basic but profound ingredients. (1) Being congruent and genuine with the client forms a safe and trusting therapeutic relationship. (2) Showing empathy for all experiences and beliefs enables the client to demystify and untangle hidden feelings and beliefs. (3) Showing unconditional positive regard allows the client to value their experiences when often they disregard feelings as silly, ridiculous, and wrong.

From Empathy to Curiosity

In order to explain the systemic ideas that could complement a humanistic orientation, let's start with a concept that is central to systemic counselling called "curiosity". Curiosity is like the idea of unconditional positive regard, which Carl Rogers defined as being attentive and sensitive to the client without passing judgement. Curiosity has a similar feel to it, trying to show the client you are focused on them supportively and non-judgementally, but instead of seeing the person and their words as isolated things out there in the world, we see their words and feelings as

DOI: 10.4324/9781003480808-3

attached to relationships. We could call this "systemic curiosity" or "system-centred counselling" because what we do is show interest in the person in connection with their relationships and environment.

It's crucial to see this difference between a stance of person-centred empathy and a stance of system-centred curiosity. Many counsellors, being excellent person-centred practitioners, miss out on the systemic effects of their therapeutic skills. In a common example, showing unconditional positive regard to a person whose parent withdraws love from them can relieve the emotional effects of the situation. But in an unforeseen result, the counsellor's empathy increases the person's opposition to their parent, and they return to therapy more frustrated. What's happening here, systemically, is that the opposition to the parent is part of the parent's reason for feeling the need to withdraw from them. As such, by amplifying the individual experience in the relationship we may have reinforced the pattern. In a more complex and systemic way, when one person in a relationship changes, usually the others in that relationship behave more rigidly until that person begins to behave like they used to, to maintain relationship stability. That is, systemic curiosity adds onto a Rogerian person-centred approach an awareness of how empathy contributes to the system of interactions. The curiosity technique is to listen to the client while not joining or reinforcing negative aspects of, in this case, their family dynamics. We may use person-centred techniques, such as probing skills and restating skills, but we orient them towards the system around the problem, asking about the responses and effects of their responses when the client interacts with other people. Let's look at some examples.

Person-Centred Approach

Client: I just feel like my mum hates me, she enjoys it when I feel crap, and this makes me SO angry.

Therapist (restating skill): You feel like your mum hates you and enjoys when you feel crap?

Client: Yes, she doesn't get what it's like for me, it's so annoying.

Therapist (probing skill): How do you experience being annoyed?

The purpose of restating and probing is to centre on the client non-judgementally, without interrupting their free expression. By taking some important part of the client's speech or experience and turning it into a question, we deepen their awareness of themselves. But this approach is not entirely free of values and is making certain kinds of judgements about what is or is not important. In the text above, there are clear choices that the counsellor is making based on a humanistic theory, such as the belief that by probing into the annoyance the client deepens their self-awareness. A system-centred approach would use curiosity towards how the annoyance is part of a pattern that keeps the presenting problem in its place.

System-Centred Approach

Client:	I just feel like my mum hates me, she enjoys it when I feel crap, and this makes me SO angry.
Therapist (restating skill):	You feel like your mum hates you and enjoys when you feel crap?
Client:	Yes, she doesn't get what it's like for me, it's so annoying.
Therapist (probing skill):	What do you do when you are annoyed? How do you show annoyance?

Moving from the client's feelings and experiences to what they do and how they show their feelings is the beginning of a systemic approach. Gianfranco Cecchin, who pioneered the use of curiosity in counselling, saw that a curious stance unravelled the interpersonal patterns that were responsible for individual mental health problems. Cecchin was not against the humanistic idea that growth comes from within but saw humanism as one of multiple ways of viewing clients' issues. Using a stance of curiosity is an orientation towards patterns rather than discrete entities like emotions or internal beliefs.

Circular Questioning

When we see the client through a person-centred lens, it is natural for us to question how the client experiences the world in the present moment. We ask the classic question, almost stereotyped by every non-counsellor, "how do you feel?". Here we probe into the felt-experience with open questions, bringing attention to the distress and insecurities that are under the surface. Person-centred therapy intensifies the present experience of the client to acknowledge it, face it, and, ultimately, to tolerate it. In this modality, the therapeutic concept of "working through the problem" means sitting with emotions empathically such that the client has fewer internal conflicts. By centring on the person and their experiences, clients feel their feelings with more acceptance and safety.

System-empathy or curiosity, on the other hand, maps out the system surrounding the feelings and problems instead of probing into the psychological experience of one person. This is done via a systemic technique called circular questioning, which acknowledges that when two or more people are in communication, each turn in the sequence of communication is part of a larger sequence or circular loop. And each response is a response to another person's response. And each response to a response is a response to another person's response. You get the idea …

Circular questioning aims to map out the interaction patterns of the family, the sibling pair, the couple, or the system that results in the problem. By asking questions about the sequence of interactions, we learn incredibly useful information that helps to make a difference in the overall pattern, changing people's emotional experiences. In straightforward terms, the technique is related to a core difficulty in systemic therapy where, instead of imagining an experience of a person, we must picture an interaction pattern.

If we cannot see the interaction pattern in front of us, how could we imagine it? Well, a circular question is a way to invite the client to reflect on and describe the sequence to you, forming a mind map from the client's perspective. For example:

Q: What does your father do when you show annoyance towards your mother?

This circular question searches for the pattern of which the problem is one event. But circular questions can be dizzying, so let's take a moment to process that question!

Q: What does your father do when you show annoyance towards your mother? ...

Here, in systemic language, we are asking a sequential question to learn about the sequence of events surrounding the problem connecting to three individuals: the client, their father, and their mother. If the client's father "does nothing" or "shouts" then we can ask clarification questions like "why does he shout when you show annoyance towards your mother?" or "when he does nothing, what does your mother think of this?". Answers to these questions allow us to slowly draw the mental map of the system that keeps the problem in place. You will see how profound these questions really are when we start to apply them to case studies.

For now, it is important to realise that circular questions are the foundation of systemic techniques because they provide the counsellor and the client(s) with a map of the relationships that create the issues that bring them to therapy. Circular questions reveal a wealth of information not attainable by individualistic approaches. In one recent case study, which was a couple's session, the two clients fell into a cyclical pattern of blame/defend ... and ... blame/defend (see Figure 2.1).

The presenting issue was described in linear and individual terms: She came with anger; he came with anxiety. I asked the wife a sequential question, "What is your anger a response to?". She said his quietness is like an attack, like how her father used quietness to ignore her when he was angry with her. I asked the

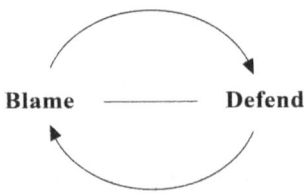

Blame ——— Defend

Figure 2.1 Blame-Defend Relationship Pattern

husband, "What is your quietness a response to?". He said he was anxious about being verbally attacked and so did not speak to his wife about his feelings. Growing up, his family did not display conflict. Raised voices constituted very serious problems. His wife saw his lack of speaking as an attack and would respond by becoming louder and by quizzing him. He saw this as an attack. The couple system was maintained through interactions of blame and defend, causing each person to suffer.

Circular questions are unusual for people and can cause pauses while people think them through. But after a few rounds of circular questioning in this situation, we arrived at an insightful moment where they began to see how their interactions were creating the problem. By avoiding being verbally attacked, he invited more verbal attacks. By attacking the silence, she was creating more silence to attack. People become stuck in conflictual interpersonal patterns by seeing only the other person's intentions and behaviours, cutting themselves out of the interaction, experiencing life as a "done to" party. Circular questions help people to realise their part in the development of their suffering. Let's say that again: circular questions help people to realise their part in the development of their suffering. We need to be careful in our understanding of power here, especially around presenting issues such as domestic violence and perpetrator responsibility, because having influence on the relationship is less possible in violent or abusive contexts. The point here to hold in mind is that, had we described him we would have named anxiety as the issue, and had we described her we would have named anger as the issue. By seeing the circularity, that the anger and anxiety kept the conflicted relationship stable, the clients developed a kind of insight not attainable with individualistic or person-centred questions—a circular insight about the patterns they were creating together. However, when violence or abuse are involved in the relationship then that needs to be addressed before considering ways to reflect on the circular interpersonal patterns.

Let's take a moment to review the types of circular questions that we could ask this couple or an individual in the couple if we were seeing one of them for counselling. John Burnham describes the circular questions at our disposal: sequential questions about the order of events like "what usually comes before or after an argument?" or "what events occur during a typical conflict?"; action questions to prompt clients into turning judgements like "she hates me" into actions through questions like "what does your partner do to show that she hates you?"; classification questions about the client's beliefs that determine how they would judge or classify the sequence of events, like "what would you call his actions towards you in this situation?" and "what beliefs do you have that guide the way you behave during arguments?"; diachronic questions ask about changes over time like "have you always argued with each other like this?" or "do the arguments differ over time? And if so, how?"; hypothetical questions ask "what if" something particular had happened or changed like "if he listened instead of responded straight away, how do you think this would influence your part in the argument?" or "if she had the same value around being compassionate during stress, what would this mean to you?"; and there are mind-reading questions that attempt to understand the logic or rationale for some actions within the sequence from another person's perspective, like "why do you think he responds to you in this way?" or "from her point of view, how do you think she experiences your silence?".

Circular questions cause people to see the problem from a different perspective. If the pattern is described as a hateful pattern and the client considers that the pattern could be described differently, they are taken out of their individual perspective into a relational perspective. Perhaps she does hate him? Perhaps she is asking for space? Perhaps this is how she responds to your pressuring need for reassurance? Perhaps your pressuring need for reassuring develops out of her need for space? By asking circular questions, the client learns new patterns for how to relate with others. And in systemic theory we call this a pattern-solution, where counselling is about unravelling relationship patterns. How the pattern is presented to you as an individual counsellor often says more about the individual than the pattern. Circular questions are the beginning to circularising the individual perspective.

Moving on with our integrative approach, there is a way to integrate circular questions with person-centred questions. Carl Rogers developed three fields of enquiry from which to base person-centred questions, which were subjective experience, objective facts, and relationships. It became apparent to systemic counsellors that subjective experience can be the focus of a circular question, and this was the first time an integration was possible between these approaches. This shift in thinking has allowed therapists to ask clients about experiences of relationship patterns, rather than just the patterns themselves, such as asking the couple, "how do you experience your husband's silence?". And we might refer to this as an internalised circular question. We are trying to understand experience as part of a process, such as by asking, "when you experience the silence as an attack, what bodily sensations do you feel?". Provided that we focus on "process" and "experience" together, we have successfully integrated the two approaches. It becomes more complex when we try to decide on which framework we see "ultimate" reality from, but for now suffice it to say that the unification of these approaches can be seen as unidirectional, for example, moving from experience to process as well as from process to experience, so asking the client something like "when you experience those sensations in your body, how do you respond to them?". It is my view that the integrative counsellor, someone who is open to multiple ideas about therapeutic change, has the luxury of not having to choose between approaches or theories or to privilege any idea above another.

Bateson's Triangle

Gregory Bateson was one of the pioneers of systemic theory and someone who closely studied the types of relationship patterns in humans and animals. He found three main types of relationship, which were symmetrical, complementary, and reciprocal (see Figure 2.2). A symmetrical relationship is when there is symmetry or sameness in the actions of two or more people or groups, usually where they mirror one another, and their interchanges consist of things like emulation

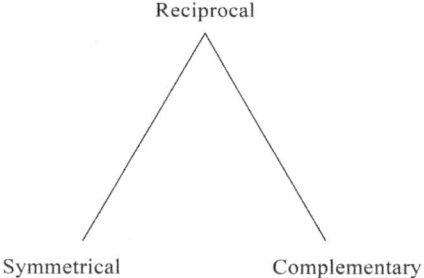

Reciprocal

Symmetrical   Complementary

Figure 2.2 Bateson's Triangle

and competition. Two boxers, two debaters, two dancers: these are symmetrical. Symmetry in relationships implies equality but not always in a useful way. For example, if a child and a parent are in a symmetrical relationship this would mean that both have equal control of the family rules. Or if two boxers from different weight classes box then one is sure to have regrets!

In contrast to symmetrical relationships, complementary relationships are those where two people have different attributes, actions, or roles but interact with some shared purpose or connection. A counsellor asks questions and the client answers. These actions *complement* one another to make up the therapeutic relationship. As we will see, complementary relationships are problematic when different roles or actions are inappropriate to the context.

Using Bateson's Triangle can help clients to identify relationship patterns that are causing them distress. It creates distinctions between relationships that are complementary, symmetrical, and reciprocal. A reciprocal relationship travels between the two extremes. They are give-and-take and can be complementary or symmetrical in different situations. When the pattern between two or more people escalates to breaking point, one person uses reciprocity by taking on the opposite style. For example, a person who is bullied until they can no longer take it changes from a complementary relationship of defending against the attacker to a symmetrical relationship of attacking the attacker. In the reverse situation, one person in an escalating symmetrical relationship might back down to prevent further escalation. As in the situation of two people in a heated debate. When the debate reaches the stage of personal insults, right before things turn hostile or even violent, one person will reciprocate and take a complementary position, agreeing to disagree. In this way, the three relationship types assist relationships in maintaining the status quo, and reciprocity brings down escalations.

In a counselling session with someone struggling to express emotions, I encouraged the client to draw the triangle and write down the significant people in her life, next to the relationship types.

Reading her diagram, the client noticed an important pattern. Her significant relationships were exclusively complementary. That is, she noticed that she was tending to give to other people and take very little for herself. The awareness gained from the technique was that it could be used to evaluate those relationships from the client's perspective, giving the client helpful insights into the presenting problem. With her counsellor, she evaluated the complementarity as appropriate for her, because she wanted me to take the lead and responsibility in asking questions, as with her manager holding authority over her complementary working role, but in other areas the complementarity caused her distress. For example, she saw her mother as needing to be cared for emotionally and she showed care to her mother by having emotional check-ins and hugs and responding to emergencies, like a parent would. The client felt unable to be cared for or understood by her mother and so her distress went unnoticed until she self-harmed and even had thoughts about committing suicide. This is what led her ultimately to therapy, because the more distress she showed, the colder her mother became, and so the client toned down her emotional signals to receive more warmth from her mother, masking the distress she was carrying.

As systemic therapists we describe this relationship between mother and daughter as a complementary pattern. In supporting the client out of a very dark place, Bateson's Triangle helped the client to evaluate her relationship boundaries with her mother. Although she worried about missing out on affection by being emotionally "louder", and by not taking the complementary role of carer for her mother's emotional needs, when the client began to seek emotional support from her mother, her mother said she appreciated the opportunity to be more of a "mum" and said she was harbouring guilt for the times she used her daughter like a therapist. It is important to remember that, in a systemic view, we do not name the mother's emotional needs as causing her daughter to be emotionally concealed, but, in a circular and relational way, mother-daughter interactions created those attributes in the two individual people, for reasons we will examine in the next section, by trapping them in a complementary pattern that was inappropriate for their relationship type: a reversal of the parent-child relationship. Clients who become carers for their carers often bring this dynamic into therapy by minimising their distress, and we can use Bateson's Triangle to explore this with the client.

A Discussion on Theory

We have so far made some sizable assumptions about what it means to experience the world and have psychological problems. In this section we will spell out as clearly as we can the ideas that are underneath the interventions discussed already.

Personality Theory

Client-centred therapy bases itself on a theory of individual personality. Rogers put forward the underlying components of personality theory and he called them "The Propositions". Rooting personality in experience, the first proposition is that every individual lives at the centre of a constantly changing world of experience. People react to the world not as the world is objectively, but in terms of their private reality, which Rogers called the perceptual field. Reactions are said to come from the whole person, as they are, with their basic tendency to develop, maintain, and enhance their psychological experience in connection with bodily states. Behaviour is therefore an outcome of goal-directed attempts to satisfy needs as they are perceived, not necessarily as they are. This means that emotions serve the function of reaching physical and social goals that attempt to enhance the experience of the individual. Counselling works by situating itself in the experience of the individual, being client-centred, understanding a person's behaviours and emotions from their internal frame of reference. Working within the limits of this internal frame, the counsellor can help the client to become aware of how their perceptions have come to define who they are and how they experience.

There is an implied systemic interpretation in personality theory in that Rogers views the organised personality of the individual as the result of interactions with the environment. Values from the environment are taken on as reality itself and these values organise how the individual experiences and values themselves. The concept of self is shaped by the interplay between experience and environment and the personality of the individual becomes more or less fixed or rigid into the self-structure. Rogers says that when personality is set, new experiences will be organised into the self-image, ignored if no relationship between the self and experience is perceived, or completely denied when the experience is inconsistent with the structure of the self. Counselling is therefore a reconstruction of the personality because, by centring on the person's experience and perceptions, they become more aware of ignored or denied experiences and can integrate them into a new sense of self, rejecting, reperceiving, and reexperiencing older parts of their personality.

Homeostasis Theory

In person-centred and humanistic theories in general, the natural tendency of the individual is to attain self-actualisation, to develop, to accept and tolerate experience, reaching their potential by evolving their personality. The systemic counterpart of the self-actualising principle, homeostasis, is the crux of a systems approach and means that individual personality and experience is a function of keeping the balance between different people in the family, the couple, the peer group, the workplace, and the society. In Chapter 1 we mentioned Bronfenbrenner who showed that individual identity is formed from the family, community, and society in which the person grows up. Homeostasis is a word for the balance between individual, family, community, and society.

Homeostasis is illustrated by the thermostat in your home, which keeps the house temperature stable using coldness from outside as information to heat up the radiators inside. This is much like our couple in the earlier section of this chapter. Emotional heat from the wife created an emotionally frozen response from the husband, often until one person became metaphorically broken or the relationship ended. Analogously to the thermostat, the couple or family might be stable in a systemic sense but have significant mental health problems where people seem to actively self-de-actualise to stay within the trappings of the relationship. The more unwell one person is, the more another learns to look after them and sacrifice their own emotional needs, perhaps even creating chronic depression or anxiety in the caring person.

In homeostasis theory, the person develops a stable sense of self, but their personality is part of multiple personalities that hang together and stabilise the couple or family system on through to stabilising the society. Social structures hang in the balance of the individuals and ecosystems they create. In fact, a society is made from people and cultures but is separate from it, in the sense that the society keeps going despite the individual people, through birth and death, constantly changing. The same is true of your body, where each of your individual cells is replaced millions and millions of times during your lifespan while your body remains intact.

WIPs and PIPs

Homeostasis and systems theory essentially notice that human systems are made from individual people and that changes in individual people trigger changes in others. Responses from one person to another preserve the homeostasis or thermostat of the system in ways that create reoccurring patterns. Karl Tomm refers to these circular patterns as "IPs" or "Interpersonal Patterns" and the two most common IPs are Wellness Interpersonal Patterns or "WIPs" and Pathologising Interpersonal Patterns or "PIPs". Karl Tomm defines a pathologising interpersonal pattern as a repeated interpersonal interaction which activates or increases negativity, pain, and suffering in one or both persons interacting, or which results in a deterioration of the relationship. With two or more clients these patterns become very clear but, within the counselling room, usually where only one person is available, we must be inventive in helping clients to recognise their IPs.

The technique is to physically draw out the interpersonal diagram with the client.

Let us take an example of a male client who came to therapy for anxiety issues. He said he had trouble with being confident in relationships and felt that significant others "treaded all over him". We drew out some of his IPs and realised that many of them were PIPs. Counsellors can start the drawing on whichever side of the interaction is chosen by the client (see Figure 2.3).

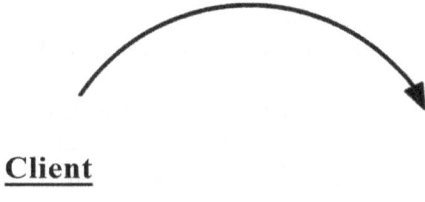

Client

Contacts girlfriend
Feels worried about the response
Does not want to argue

Figure 2.3 Half an Interpersonal Pattern

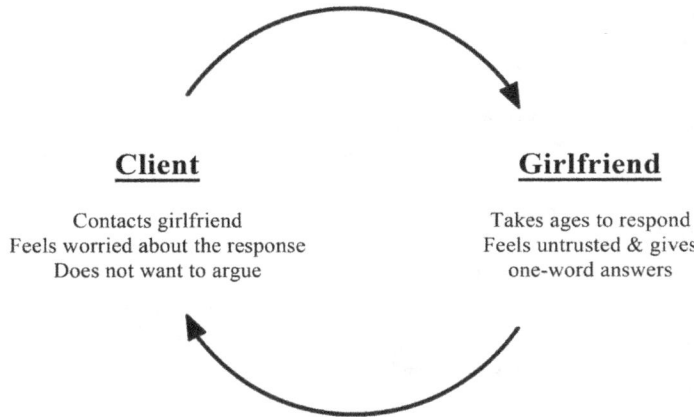

Client   **Girlfriend**

Contacts girlfriend   Takes ages to respond
Feels worried about the response   Feels untrusted & gives
Does not want to argue   one-word answers

Figure 2.4 A Whole Interpersonal Pattern

After we have a start to the diagram, we ask the client to draw the response within the interpersonal pattern (Figure 2.4).

Then we are curious about each word, thought, feeling, and experience. For example, we ask the question, "How do you know that your girlfriend felt frustrated by your message?". In our example, the client filled in the detail that his girlfriend texted one-word answers. At this stage, like in person-centred therapy, we map out the client's experience of the interaction with curiosity and circular questions. For example, we might start the next phase of the diagram by asking a sequential question like "When your girlfriend showed frustration at your messages, how did you respond?". The answers are then drawn or written onto the diagram. Karl Tomm has a very careful way of drawing interpersonal patterns but for the purposes of integrative counselling we suggest viewing the essential point as helping the client to map out their difficulties in a circular way, whether you use arrows or other notations. For instance, with younger children, we might ask them to draw the interactions into a comic book or storyboard or for adolescents and adults we might draw the cycles in a table (see Table 2.1).

In this example, the diagramming helped the client to see that his confidence level was tied up with his complementary interpersonal patterns. Thinking of ways to shift the pattern from a pathologising pattern to a wellness pattern affected positive change in his relationship. He explored the idea that starting the interaction with a question about feelings was a way for him to subtly show his worries about his partner's mood. Picking up on this unspoken communication, new information came to him from his girlfriend who said she often felt attacked by his text messages that asked how she was doing because they implied that she was moody or frustrated. What fascinated me here was that both people felt trapped in the other person's invitation for conflict. It is very common that people feel positioned by others until they become aware of the circularity involved, like our client, who

Table 2.1 Client Interpersonal Patterns

Client	Interaction	Girlfriend
Initiates contact by text message, "How are you?" Feels worried about negative responses Does not want to argue		Takes a while to respond Feels frustrated and messages back with one-word answers
Confidence drops Feels defensive Thinks "I make everything worse" Withdraws, stops messaging		Impatient Sends critical text messages "Why have you gone silent?" Withdraws, stops messaging

figured out that his defences and her attacks, together, were creating his lower levels of confidence. A person-centred therapist might see this as the client becoming aware of his role in undermining his confidence.

When using IP diagrams with clients, we can consider ways of generating "WIPs" or Wellness Interpersonal Patterns, which Karl Tomm describes as repeated patterns that generate and sustain health in the relationship. The client in this section already began to imagine ways of moving from a PIP to a WIP in his relationship, for instance by imagining ways to begin the interaction differently or by responding differently when one-word answers evoke low self-confidence in him. Tomm refers to these circular questions as "interventive" questions, because the questions are a form of intervention. They set up a circular perspective that changes how the client views the problem.

As the cliché goes, when looking at an individual problem like anxiety and low self-worth, we should remind ourselves that it takes two to tango. With one client in the room, systemic counsellors support individuals to reflect on their part in creating pathologising interpersonal patterns to support them in making shifts towards wellness patterns. With two or more people in the room, we explore the interpersonal patterns in real time by using creative methods like Bateson's Triangle or circular questions. We know from Cooper, Elliot et al., and King et al. that client-centred counselling reduces distress, depression, and worry by offering therapeutic relationships to clients based on empathy, unconditional positive regard, and congruence. The work of Alan Carr has shown that systemic approaches work with the same individual problems, and this chapter has attempted to integrate person-centred ideas with systemic ideas to demonstrate the usefulness of a system-centred approach. Now we will move into a different counselling modality to continue to underscore systemic ideas across the spectrum of integrative approaches.

Further Reading

Bateson, G. (1972). *Steps to an ecology of mind*. San Francisco: Chandler.

Burnham, J. (1986). *Family therapy*. London: Routledge.

Carr, A. (2014a). The evidence-base for family therapy and systemic interventions for child-focused problems. *Journal of Family Therapy, 36*, 107–157.

Carr, A. (2014b). The evidence-base for couple therapy, family therapy and systemic interventions for adult-focused problems. *Journal of Family Therapy, 36*, 158–194.

Cecchin, G. (1987). Hypothesising, circularity and neutrality revisited. An invitation to curiosity. *Family Process, 24*(1), 15–25.

Cooper, M (2010). *Essential research findings in counselling and psychotherapy: The facts are friendly*. London: Sage Publications LTD.

Elliott, R., Greenberg, L., & Lietaer, G. (2004). Research on experiential psychotherapies. In M. Lambert (Ed.), *Bergin and Garfield's handbook of psychotherapy and behaviour change* (5th ed., pp. 493–539). New York: Wiley.

King, M., Sibbald, B., Ward, E., Bower, P., Lloyd, M., Gabbey, M., et al. (2000). Randomised control trials of non-directive counselling, cognitive-behaviour therapy and usual general practitioner care in the management of depression as well as mixed anxiety and depression in primary care. *Health Technology Assessment, 19*(1), 1–83.

Rogers, C. (2020). *Client-centred therapy* (70th ed.). London: Robinson.

Tomm, K. M. (1991). Beginnings of a "HIPs and PIPs" approach to psychiatric assessment. *The Calgary Participator, 1*(2), 21–24.

Chapter 3

Psychosystemic Counselling

The advent of the talking cure was a phenomenal moment in the history of psychology. Sigmund Freud and his mentor Josef Breuer were physicians who treated patients with very peculiar symptoms such as those of Anna O. She, despite having no clear and obvious physical health problems, was suffering from hallucinations and paralysis of her arm and leg. With few medical options at his disposal, Breuer decided to talk with Anna each day about her symptoms and noticed that not only were they predominantly connected to psychological worries but that releasing the anxious thoughts caused her symptoms to vanish. The term "talking therapy" came out of this case study and gave rise to Freud's interest in psychotherapy in general.

Now the case of Anna O. has been shown to be fabricated by Breuer and Freud. Anna most likely did have physical health problems and was most likely not fully cured, as both authors had attested to. This poses an uncomfortable problem for this chapter because we are going to look in some detail at the theories that were inspired by this landmark case knowing full-well that dishonesty was part of the messy beginning of talking therapies. Our approach will be to tell you about the field of psychodynamic counselling and then to redescribe it from a systemic perspective.

After the case of Anna O., when Freud later investigated psychosomatic problems, he found an interesting insight from the client's response to the therapist. The client showed a tendency to play out distressing feelings and behavioural patterns with their therapist that had their ultimate origins in childhood. By noticing how the client transferred onto the therapist fears, anxieties, hatred, and other emotions, Freud unravelled those interactions through questions that would turn out to be repeated patterns from the client's earliest relationships, usually their relationship with a parent.

Transference and Countertransference

The concept of transference refers to moments where the client redirects unconscious feelings, unconscious fears, and unconscious emotions from past relationships onto the counsellor. The client transfers the unconscious fear of judgement from their father or the unconscious anxiety towards their mother when talking

DOI: 10.4324/9781003480808-4

about emotions. All relationships contain some form of transference, but the therapeutic relationship is special in evoking the strongest and most relevant unconscious feelings regarding the client's psychological problems. As counsellors, we highlight transference in the words and actions of the client.

Here are some extracts from a counselling session for us to consider how words and actions signify transference. As the counsellor, we ask ourselves what previous experiences might the client be transferring onto us with these statements or actions?

Counselling Session Extract

"It's hard for me to be vulnerable in front of you. Maybe someone can use it against me".

Client rubs their arms and self-soothes when saying the above comment.

"I can't show the emotion because I feel like I have to be the brave one, like you'll think of me as weak".

A psychodynamic analysis of this transcript determines that the client is transferring onto the counsellor a lack of trust and safety in his care towards her vulnerability and she unconsciously self-soothes, jokes, or denies experiences of vulnerability. Because the client is unaware of their transference they will usually deny or ignore memories of having experienced that feeling in other relationships. Part of the force behind the Freudian revolution was the significance in noticing that when the client's transference is highlighted to them, they begin to experience the counsellor with fresh eyes and gain insight into the workings of their unconscious needs.

While de Maat and colleagues have demonstrated the effectiveness of long-term psychoanalytic therapy, interpreting the unconscious needs of clients comes with an important warning. Early systems theory was partly promoted by therapists because it joined the anti-Freudian movement in which challenging a therapist's power to determine how a client was interpreted was viewed as an ethical step forwards. Writers such as Todd Dufresne summarise the arguments against some psychodynamic concepts by referring to how they anoint the therapist as being all-knowing and all-defining. This promotes narcissism, sexism, and pessimism while many strict Freudians remain wilfully inattentive to social context when viewing the client's part in the transference but not their own.

Context

The systemic counsellor accepts the observable facts of psychoanalysis but understands them differently, sidestepping any power-hungriness by referring to the idea of context. A context is a frame that gives things their meaning. For instance, if a person laughs nearby another person it does not take on a meaning until situated in a context. Was the laugh in the context of the person's fashion choice? Was it in response to a joke? Did the laugh come from a stranger when viewing another stranger? Were they being asked out on a date? Was the laugh evoking a context of hatred or a context of connection? A systems perspective sees transference as being drawn out by the context of counselling, linked with how the interpersonal patterns develop into relationships.

Gregory Bateson noticed that transference comes from the client's patterns-of-relating within a context, sometimes the context of childhood, the context of being cared for, and the context of authority. In fact, in his book *Mind and Nature* he said, "the patterns and experiences of childhood are built into me" (p. 13). In this sense, a person's parents, say, their father, are a context that gives meaning to the relationship between father and child. When a fatherly context is evoked, perhaps by consulting a male therapist, a male teacher, or a male boss, the client demonstrates their patterns-of-relating through transference. In the context of fatherly or parental relationships people are transferring past learning from this context onto the counsellor. It is this context of care and authority that evokes the transferred patterns of relating, and, as such, if we shift the context then we shift the meaning and experience of the client.

Systemic theory places human systems inside ecosystems, and describes how they are self-corrective by using feedback and circular causations. Interactions between people stabilise their relationships with continuous feedback loops and responsiveness. Context happens when a pattern is the same over time in a particular situation. For example, if I repeatedly receive love from a female caregiver then I begin to enter into interactions with female caregivers with this expectation. I have learned a context for ways of interacting with female caregivers. In the counselling room the client plays out their learned patterns of interactions, their contexts, or ways of making meaning, which is understood as a form of contextual transference because a context for the relationship is being transferred from client to counsellor. Using the machine metaphor, Bateson says that our relationship experiences encode learning and that psychological growth takes place when new relationship-coding takes place. If the client learns to experience care within the therapeutic relationship, they are more able to interact with others in ways that generate healthier interpersonal patterns. This is shown by looking at the words from clients later in the counselling, highlighting any change in what the client is transferring into the relationship. For example, the client from earlier in this chapter said in a later counselling session:

"I am showing more emotion around you than I thought I would".

"I have started doing that more, being vulnerable around you, it's become a bit more okay now".

The changes expressed in these quotes are consistent with psychodynamic and systemic thinking. They highlight that the client has shifted from transferring a lack of hope and safety in being vulnerable to a position of comfort in being emotional.

Relational Reflexivity

Instead of overcoming the unconscious experience of, say, parental rejection or abusive strictness, a systemic counsellor works with the pattern in the room, seeing themselves as part of the pattern. One effort in working with the pattern between counsellor and client was made by John Burnham with a systemic technique called "relational reflexivity". Here the counsellor intentionally focuses the attention on the therapeutic relationship, asking the client about their experience of the relationship and the hopes they have.

John gives the example of working with avoidance. He noticed his internal voice saying that the client was changing the subject every time she approached an important issue. Now a transference-oriented counsellor would focus the client on their avoidance or, in a systemic framing, on their half of the pattern, whereas the relationally reflexive therapist focuses on the client's experience of the whole pattern with the counsellor. Instead of the psychodynamic question, "how do you experience talking about a difficult issue?", he asked the systemic question, "who do you think avoids it more ... me or you?". To his surprise, the client experienced John as the avoidant one, as he was saying things like "You don't have to talk about this now" to reassure the client, who found him to be the one that needed rescuing from the difficult subject!

By asking questions about the relationship pattern, from the client's perspective, and by sharing experiences from your perspective, the transference is explored as a circular pattern, rather than as something fixed inside the client. Freud himself noticed this fact, that counsellors begin to take on the role of the frustrated parent or the avoidant caregiver, and he termed this "countertransference". In the modern psychoanalytic definition of this word, this would mean any feelings the counsellor has towards the client, and often highlights the counsellor's own relationship history.

Relational reflexivity asks questions about the therapeutic relationship to co-create and encode new learning or experiences of the therapist with the client. Asking questions such as "How would you like this therapy to go?" or "What do we both do to contribute to your fear of showing vulnerability?" is a way to coordinate the resources of the therapist and the client for developing the therapeutic relationship. But an issue arises with the word "reflexive" that we should unpack a little more.

Reflexivity often gets confused with reflection and this blurs the underlying ideas. Reflection is a mirroring or a showing back. Self-reflection is looking back on the self and is constituted by breaking down the self into aspects like habits, personality, childhood, and behaviour, and pausing to process these aspects of the self. Reflexivity stretches beyond reflection to uncover what learning takes place from reflection. That is, self-reflexivity is when the act of personal reflection creates a new way of seeing or understanding the self. We can apply this to relational reflexivity. This is not an act of reflecting back but of learning from reflecting back on aspects of the therapeutic relationship, including those aspects that are desired rather than actualised. Burnham's simplest example is in the notion of "questions about questions" in which he describes relational reflexivity as asking questions about the questions and practices in therapy. For instance, "When I ask about your family, is this more or less useful?" or "What types of questions do you prefer at this moment, questions about emotions, questions about family, questions about work, or other types of questions?". The insight here is that clients begin to realise that they can actively participate in building and developing relationships, giving them more freedom from old patterns of relating. This is the new relationship coding that Bateson speaks of.

Second-Order Cybernetics

The science of systems was called cybernetics by Norbert Wiener, meaning a "steersman" of a system, like the captain of a ship. But he and other systems theorists originally did not notice that observers are part of the systems they describe. It took people like Von Foerster to develop the idea of the observer being part of the system, which he called second-order cybernetics. Thus, when I describe the pattern between client and family, or client and me, for example, I am doing so from a perspective, not an objective viewpoint.

What psychotherapy has missed since the time of Freud, particularly in now-taboo theories like "everything human beings do is symbolically about sex", is that the observer is part of the system. Is it possible, for example, that Freud's maleness influenced his way of connecting cigars with penises? Many anti-Freudian books have claimed exactly this! (Although, beyond the grave, Freud has argued that the anti-Freudians merely confirm his view that metaphorical fathers are to be rebelled against if their children are to be successful!)

The point is that, as a counsellor, my background, history, life experiences, values, and beliefs significantly distort, change, and shape what I see in the world around me. When I respond to the world, I am bringing a set of relationships and meanings that correspond to my political ideas, personal feelings, and professional views. A systemic counsellor is seeing their interventions as part of creating contexts and meaning with clients. One cannot avoid their words having influence and so we need techniques to limit the counsellor's bias—or countertransference—on the client. Taking a second-order position creates special ways of intervening that are novel in systemic work. These techniques seek to address the therapy system in a way that generates change for the rules governing the system, and relational reflexivity is one such second-order technique. We will discuss more in subsequent chapters.

The Structure of Mind

Relational reflexivity relies on openness and transparency in therapy, and this can be hard work when clients have learned from contexts of abuse, neglect, and other difficult situations, the interpersonal patterns of withholding emotions and experiences. Understanding why people withhold emotions is made possible by diving deeper into Freud's work, particularly into his model of the mind.

Freud asserted the theory of the pleasure principle to be what underpins all human behaviour, including expressing emotions. His view was essentially Darwinian, considering how evolution shaped human genetics to want to survive.

He said that things that benefit survival are experienced as pleasurable and things that restrain survival are felt as pain, or unpleasure. In this theory, culture is seen as a by-product of universal needs.

In Austria the national dish is Wiener Schnitzel, in Hungary it's Goulash, in France it's Pot-au-Feu, and in England it's fish and chips. Whatever the specific culture is around food, you would do well to predict that any human population that survives today would have specific customs around eating. Freud proposed that behaviour is driven by these universal needs, or instincts, which, when not met appropriately, are responsible for pathology, neurosis, and general discontent in child and adult life. Essentially, the physical energy that drives the instincts becomes stored in the mind, unconsciously, which is why he called the theory psychodynamic theory, to fit in with the physicists who used the word "dynamic" to think about energy systems.

In psychodynamic theory, the natural tendency of individuals is to attain pleasure but of course one encounters an often-hostile reality in which psychological needs are left unmet or even damaged. Freud posited that the earlier development of the mind, which he called the Id, driven by the pleasure principle, must give way to a more conscious part of the mind called the Ego, which is governed by the real-world reality principle. These competing parts of the mind, one supplying our psychological energy—our psychodynamics—for what we unrealistically want and need, the other supplying energy for what we realistically must tolerate, led to internalised rules about how to be in the world in relation to meeting our needs. This third part of psychological development was termed the Superego. Not because it had superpowers but because it supervises the ego and is our internalised system of rules for governing between our needs and our reality.

Defence Mechanisms

It was mostly out of the transference relationship where Sigmund Freud is said to have discovered the unconscious mind for the development of his psychodynamic theory. Here the unconscious is not seen but inferred by looking at how people behave when they show a lack of insight into their behaviour and the reasons for their behaviour. Distressed people might be incoherent in their speech, hallucinate, or become phobic of harmless things, being unable to account for why these abnormalities are happening to them. This fundamental observation in psychoanalysis led Freud and his followers to see the unconscious as a source of energy for disturbed behaviour resulting from previous and most likely troubling experiences. This window into the unconscious grew into the theory of psychoanalysis. A healthy person, according to Freud, has a strong ego. They can satisfy the needs of their id without trespassing too much on the rules of the superego, able to face the reality in front of them.

In psychodynamic theory, a psychological defence is a mechanism or strategy by which a person seeks, consciously or unconsciously, to protect themselves from real or perceived painful or threatening attacks to their ego. When the id has unmet needs, they surface as defence mechanisms by distorting conscious reality as the client perceives it.

A common defence mechanism is repression, in which a person who has experienced painful feelings that were intolerable at a previous time tries to avoid re-experiencing those feelings. An anxious person may have experienced difficult separations from caregivers. This could relate to work, neglect, culture, illness, or death. The id's need to be comforted by that person becomes energised and amplified significantly, causing a great deal of distress at the time that may be very painful to tolerate. Fast-forwarding to the person's adulthood, if the energy pent up in unconscious separation anxiety surfaces due to a new intimate relationship, then the person may repress the fear of separation by—again, unconsciously—emotionally distancing from that person or becoming overwhelmingly dependable. Emotional distance and dependableness are defences when they serve the function of hiding the unconscious fear of separation.

Malan's Triangle

Psychodynamic counsellors support clients to overcome defence mechanisms by helping them to notice the defence mechanism, experience the anxiety, and recover the hidden feeling. The most powerful technique for this comes from the late David Malan of the Tavistock Clinic in London and is called "Malan's Triangle". (Actually, it is plural as there are two triangles, but we needn't worry about that for now!)

The triangle is based on the idea that the defence mechanism is able to hide a feeling by creating anxiety if a situation arises that recalls the past painful feeling. The anxiety then creates a behaviour that covers over, unconsciously, the hidden feeling. For instance, when someone wants to hide from their awkwardness, they joke; when someone wants to hide from their anxiety, they project it onto someone else and treat that someone else as if they were anxious; when someone's superego whispers into the unconscious part of their ego that it is socially unacceptable to be violent, they hide their aggression in falsely passive comments that cause aggression in others. Each of us uses denial, repression, projection, and displacement to make sure that hurtful feelings remain hidden from our conscious awareness though they are experienced and carried in the body. Buried feelings usually come back to haunt. The client usually comes to therapy when their defence mechanisms cause pathology.

We can use Malan's Triangle to develop the client's awareness of their unconscious feelings. We start by noticing a defence mechanism such as humour, rationalisation, or projection. For instance, a client who had a painful separation from her mother when aged 8–12 has now moved from home to university. When asked about her feelings she says, "I'm fine. I don't miss her [mum] or anything. I've been lonely, a bit, but … Oh I forgot to tell you, I have a new cat!"

Here the client uses several defence mechanisms; for example, she denies the emotional impact of change and separation and she represses feelings using humour, distraction, and storytelling. In noticing the defence, the counsellor maintains the relationship as the top priority and rolls with the defences, listening to the story about the cat before bringing the topic of separation back into the room, communicating "we can face this". The counsellor highlights the defences with curiosity, "it feels like a choice to talk about the cat or the loneliness and separation from your mum". Psychodynamically, if defence mechanisms are removed the client has more ability to face reality, manage separation, and increase resilience through change rather than pseudo-resilience that leads to loneliness, depression, and anxiety. With this client, mapping out Malan's Triangle (Figure 3.1) helped her to understand the defence mechanism. In using this tool, the client began to cry, saying that she was upset and scared that she does not have her mum as her "emotional safety net".

The triangle we have been discussing is called the "triangle of conflict" because it represents the inner conflict of the client. The second triangle is called the "triangle of insight" (see Figure 3.2) because it enables psychodynamic counsellors to make links with the client about their inner conflicts and their past and present experiences. These links are known in psychodynamic language as interpretations. The first interpretation is between what a person describes in their current situation and a past event or relationship. The second interpretation is between the current situation and the counselling relationship or the transference. And the third interpretation is between the client's past and the present situation with the counsellor, which is the transference. Using the complete triangle to make an interpretation is what Freud referred to as a psychodynamic construction.

For example, with our client we might ask how her current separation from her mother is like her past childhood separation from her mother. If the client feels

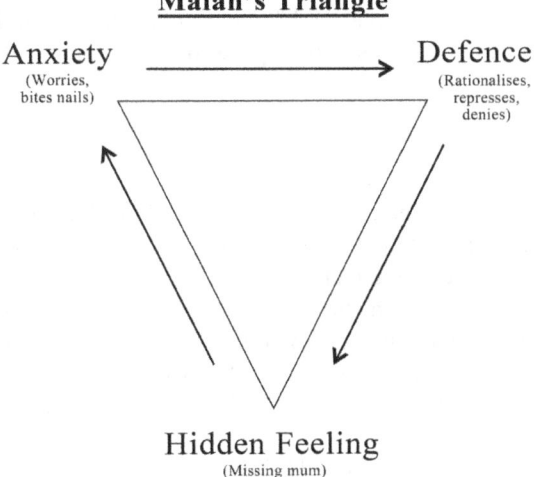

Malan's Triangle

Anxiety ⟶ Defence
(Worries, bites nails) (Rationalises, represses, denies)

Hidden Feeling
(Missing mum)

Figure 3.1 Malan's Triangle

Triangle of Insight

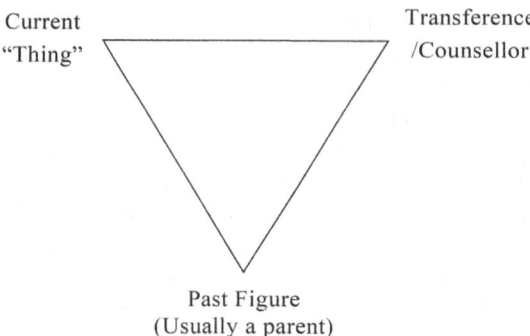

Current "Thing"

Transference /Counsellor

Past Figure
(Usually a parent)

Figure 3.2 Triangle of Insight

unable to express emotions to me as the counsellor, we might ask if the barrier in the counsellor relationship is similar to past relationships where she feels unable to express emotions. Making links in a tentative way helps the client to gain insight.

A systemic view sees the same observations as the psychodynamic counsellors do, that people hide from their feelings, become phobic of buttons and doorknobs, and people believe in delusions like believing the wind is a ghost haunting their family, but systemic theory has a different picture of what is going on. The work of Gregory Bateson showed that mental health disorders such as panic disorder, with which our client above was diagnosed, happen in communication processes. Like in psychoanalysis, these processes are seen as non-conscious but are more observable when you put two or more people in communication with one another. In this example, the client denied that she was missing her mother, minimising her feelings with phrases like "it's not the end of the world" and "I don't mind", and when she did begin to feel some of the loneliness, she repressed the feelings with humour and storytelling.

Reframing

The systemic counterpart of the pleasure principle, which we named in Chapters 1 and 2 as the principle of homeostasis, is that human nature does not work by seeking pleasure but by keeping a balance between the elements in their social environment. As we have seen, the thermostat keeps the house temperature stable but the colder the outside, the hotter the radiators must be. Analogously, the client might be stable in a relational sense but have significant mental health problems, seeming to an outside observer to actively seek displeasure or even pain in order to maintain the status quo of the relationship.

The psychoanalytic concept of insight has profoundly shaped the practice of psychotherapy for the last century. Unconscious of our inner drives, we are enslaved to routine habits and psychological defence mechanisms that allow us to cope with the world. Finding out that we reject people we love because we have been trau-matically rejected as children, gaining some semblance of emotional control at the cost of having hollow and anxious relationships, opens our eyes to different ways of seeing and being in the world. Systemic theory puts forward a relational form of the concept of insight less attached to internalised energy systems yet founded on the same observation that people can change their habits when they become aware of the mechanisms that stabilise them. Systemic insight is connected to the word "frame" and reframing is a technique that brings it about.

The basic idea is that relationship patterns stabilise in relation to a psychologi-cal frame, which is the context for a person's experience. How people frame their relationships or how they define their relationships translates into meanings and feelings about the other person and justifies their part in the interpersonal pattern. Defence mechanisms are therefore describable in terms of habituated circular pat-terns in which emotions become repressed. For example, if a mother and daughter non-consciously define their relationship as something like "a biological relation for practical support where difficult emotions cannot be expressed", a change in the definition of the relationship would get them out of their entrenched patterns and defence mechanisms. In this current definition, if the daughter becomes much more emotionally needy of her parent, it is likely that her mother will withdraw emotional support more extremely, and thus maintain the overall definition of the relationship. The change in the defence mechanism had no overall change in the relationship pattern. This is often what clients mean when we support them to make a change and they point out that changing themselves can feel futile if others don't change.

Let's develop Karl Tomm's model of interpersonal patterns by helping the cli-ent to think about the frame of the relationship. We can ask the client something like: how would you define your relationship with your mum? And the client might say "Detached Mother-Daughter Relationship" (see Figure 3.3). This definition is

Detached Mother-Daughter Relationship

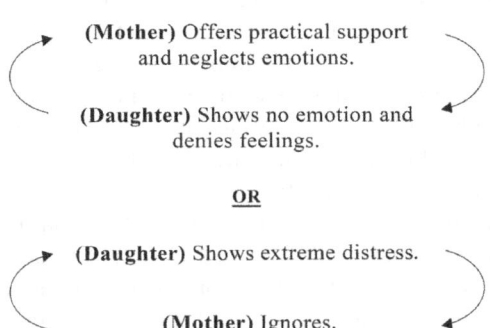

Figure 3.3 Detached Mother-Daughter Relationship

the context for the actions of the participants in the relationship. It helps to explain where the defence mechanisms come from.

Though the two cycles in Figure 3.3 seem very different in terms of the felt experience of the two people, systemically it is the same complementary pattern and is maintaining the overarching frame of their relationship.

Systemic Change

To understand the nuts and bolts of reframing one must take on some new and systemic ideas about change. If a person wishes to change their deeply ingrained habits, they can create behavioural changes in their routine. For example, someone who wants to lose weight might eat fewer calories or increase their exercise. Behavioural change is called a first-order change and for many people first-order change is enough to change the habit. The thermostat metaphor we used earlier is a good illustration of first-order change. The sun comes out or a blizzard hits town, but either way, the home remains a comfortable 20 or so degrees Celsius because any change in temperature evokes a change in the overall heating and air-conditioning systems (broken boiler not included). If you want to change the temperature of the home then you need to change the rules of the system or the setting on the thermostat, say, to 18 degrees Celsius, and this is a second-order change. The key to why most people struggle to change a habit is because they make first-order changes. That is, they may eat less and exercise more for one week and then overcompensate with sofa time and snacking the next week, thus maintaining homeostasis overall.

Systemic views on defence mechanisms are that defence mechanisms are an enactment of learned patterns-of-relating. Personality is our habituated patterns of relating and experiencing within different contexts. This accounts for why we become completely different and even contradictory people in different contexts. Thus, systemic techniques aim to change the frame of reference that is hurting the person and their relationships. If I live by the unwritten rule that I cannot show emotion to caregivers, then I will ultimately be unhappy. The nature-nurture debate raises its head here. Because the question arises as to whether people are fundamentally different on a genetic level. A systemic counsellor needn't get caught up in this debate; a person may be more genetically "wired" to become angry when she perceives threat, for example, but counselling may redefine how she perceives threat and so she runs into fewer problems of anger during her life situations. Reframing means to place the events or problems into a new framework or context, thereby changing its entire meaning. Reframing leaves the facts as they are.

The theory of change in systems theory begins with thinking about circularity and researchers such as Baucom have shown the effectiveness of reducing individual pathology through couple or system-oriented interventions. This is because problems arise from circular interactions between people. But the context or reason for this interaction is that a frame hangs over each turn in the social interaction, defining the relationship and generating habituated patterns. Working on the definition of the relationship, on the rules of the interaction, creates a change in the system, or a second-order change. For example, by working on the client's defence mechanisms, and mapping out the interpersonal patterns that create them, the client from earlier reframed how her mother was attempting to parent. In fact, the practical support her mother offered was attempting to create a context of care. As the client perceived things differently, she was more able to access her mum's support and address the need to share more on an emotional level. A psychodynamic counsellor might describe these changes in language related to the id, ego, and superego, and researchers such as de Maat et al., Leichsenring et al., and Westen et al. have proven the case for psychodynamic therapies being effective, but both systemic and psychodynamic approaches are working to a similar outcome here and the difference may sometimes be in the description, other times the techniques. Viewing a client's problem from a psychosystemic perspective means taking on the ideas and observations from a psychodynamic approach, including transference, the unconscious mind, and defence mechanisms, while describing them and intervening with them in a systemic and relational way.

Further Reading

Bateson, G. (1980). *Mind and nature. A necessary unity.* New York: Bantam Books.

Baucom, D. H., Belus, J. M., Adelman, C. B., Fischer, M. S., & Paprocki, C. (2014). Couple-based interventions for psychopathology: A renewed direction for the field. *Family Process Journal, 53,* 445–461. doi:10.1111/famp.12075.

Burnham, J. (2005). *Relational reflexivity: A tool for socially constructing therapeutic relationships.* London: Karnac Books.

de Maat, S., de Jonghe, F., Schoevers, R., & Dekker, J. (2009). The effectiveness of long-term psychoanalytic therapy: A systematic review of empirical studies. *Harvard Review of Psychiatry, 17,* 1–23. doi:10.1080/16073220902742476.

Freud, S. (1977). An outline of psychoanalysis. In J. Strachey (Ed.), *The standard edition of the complete psychological works of Sigmund Freud* (Vol. 23, pp. 139–207). London: Hogarth Press.

Leichsenring, F., & Rabung, S. (2008). Effectiveness of long-term psychodynamic psychotherapy: A meta-analysis. *Journal of the American Medical Association, 300,* 1551–1565.

Malan, D. (1995). *Individual psychotherapy and the science of psychodynamics.* Oxford: Butterworth-Heinemann

Watzlawick, P., Weakland, J. W., & Fisch, R. (1974). *Change.* New York: W.W. Norton & Company.

Westen, D., Novotny, C. A., & Thompson-Brener, H. (2004). The empirical status of the empirically supported psychotherapies: Assumptions, findings and reporting in controlled clinical trials. *Psychological Bulletin, 130*(4), 631–633.

Wiener, N. (1948). *Cybernetics; or control and communication in the animal and the machine.* London: Wiley.

Chapter 4

Family Counselling

Before the 1940s, psychotherapy was ignorant of family therapy and systemic thinking, although it did attempt to treat some psychological problems with family interventions. This early footprint into family therapy caused a variety of problems because the therapists, having borrowed their concepts from psychoanalysis, were seeing families as collections of individuals whose needs were isolated and internal to themselves. This led to confusion and in many situations heightened conflict. Now, in the decades that followed, partly because of the development of attachment theory and the scientific acknowledgement of how individual problems stem from relationships, people such as Murray Bowen and, much later, Virginia Satir began talking about the family as an "emotional unit", bringing in the idea that families are close-knit groups whose individual parts (the family members) collaborate to stabilise the family system. In this chapter we describe the key concepts from family therapy and demonstrate how to adapt them for counselling individual clients.

Family Lifecycles

When family therapy became theorised within psychotherapy, people immediately noticed that family stabilisation, or family homeostasis, was responsible for a great deal of the suffering that flooded its way into the clinic. Individuals were not simply broken personalities in need of fixing. Clients were caught in a web of interpersonal patterns with other family members where inexplicable and distressing behaviour served a complex systemic function.

The well-known family therapist Jay Haley used the idea of functionalism to describe families in that problems were seen as serving the function of keeping family relationships together. Carter and McGoldrick in the 1980s moved this idea forward to show how functioning in a family was constantly challenged and disrupted by the pressurising need for the family to grow within the social context. They showed that families were not static but ever-changing entanglements of people. Families hold together emotional bonds over time by frequently but nonconsciously renegotiating relationships.

DOI: 10.4324/9781003480808-5

Carter and McGoldrick discovered something that now seems obvious. As with many advances in human thinking and science! They discovered several common stages of family development that cause the family to evolve and renegotiate relationships, creating sometimes-disastrous personal problems. Family stages of development were called lifecycles to compare the development of the family with the order in nature. Like plants and animals, families have a beginning, a series of changes, and, in a certain sense, a death. Like animals and evolution in general, what we choose to call the start and end of the process is basically random. Lifecycles are defined as circular and predictable events that change the status and internal dynamics of a family. Societal, biological, and cultural life events cause families to change their interpersonal patterns, and interpersonal patterns are the foundation of psychological wellbeing. Some transitions are biologically determined, and others are determined by society and culture. Carter and McGoldrick summarise the transitions in the following way:

Courtship, early relationships, forming a couple
Early commitment, partnership/marriage
Birth of children, becoming a parent, generativity
Middle years, family with growing children
Adolescence and "launching" children
Retirement and older-age families

If we consider where interpersonal patterns come from, those circular ways in which we engage others, it is from our family, the school of contexts for much of our social development. In our family we learn how to talk with others, show affection, respond to criticism, deal with embarrassment, express anger, support those in need, and challenge immoral actions. Our ways of greeting friends, our social attitudes, and the emotions that colour our experiences are learned and practised at home. If the family was stable, if it did not change with time, we would likely be set into our roles without much strain. But this is an impossible reality. At some point, for example, someone in the family will change something, such as forming a new intimate relationship. At this lifecycle point, the role that person took in the family must change, if only because their availability for that role is lower or involves having someone new in the family.

Being in a couple system, which is a lifecycle stage, means forming a relationship where things such as commitment and belonging are defined within the boundaries of a new "us". If we then have children, say, which is another lifecycle stage, this redefines "us" as parents as well as being a couple. What worked as an interaction pattern in the couple no longer works as an interaction pattern as parents. Romance is less of a priority; nappies need changing, after all!

The man, for argument's sake, might see the mother "still" as the girlfriend, and experience her in this context. Her lower availability to show him affection is heard within the context of "girlfriend" or "wife", thus creating a response from him within that context. If he is from a family where challenge is acceptable, he expresses tension and, through the feedback loops, he learns that his partner is acting out of a parental context, not only a girlfriend context. Here he would be encouraged to join his partner in the new definition of their relationship. If he is from a family where conflict is passive, he may withdraw more. Or he may become angry. Or he may resent the child.

Psychological problems are often created by the effects of healthy development on important relationships. Adolescence, for example, which culturally becomes drowned in hormone-talk, is often problematic not because hormones cause the teenager to withdraw more to their bedroom, but because the response to this withdrawal is to raise the anxiety of the parent who knocks loudly on the door. Instead of the adolescent being viewed as developing more independence, the withdrawal is responded to as a problem to solve. Through the knocking, the ignoring, the knocking louder, the shouting, and the shouting back, a common systemic problem of chase and withdraw arises; a cat-and-mouse escalation, serving the function of stabilising the old relationship at the cost of the parent and child's wellbeing in the new situation. But the child is no longer ten years old. The relationship must change.

Family Observation

Imagine a set of parents and their teenage daughter who has recently turned 14. What are the rules governing this system or relationship? They may be things like "parents monitor children's behaviour", "parents expect their daughter to come down for meals and tidy her room". But when the child becomes older and more independent, the monitoring and expectations to be part of the family might pull the child towards the family while her friendships, social norms, and developmental age might pull her more towards having privacy, separation from the family, and spending time on social media with peers. Often families notice this change as a first-order change. That is, the child is perceived as needing to be monitored, to come down for meals, and so on, in the old frame. Seeing these behavioural changes in the child under the same child-like frame means the parents will further insist on following the child-like rules and may even start to seriously consider if they are developing a mental health disorder. So, the parents step up the monitoring of their young person and, as we all know, she responds vehemently with frustration, increased demands for privacy, and disconnection from her family. Because relationships are dynamic and not static, most families learn to change the rules of their system slowly over time, being reciprocal before things reach breaking point. Perhaps friends say, "she's just being a teenager, just leave her to it" and the family begins to reframe their daughter from a child frame to a young-adult frame. This second-order change was needed for the family to survive the lifecycle. Transitional phases are where many emotional problems develop in children and in adults.

It has been fascinating to train as a systemic psychotherapist and be invited to sit and watch ordinary families going about their daily lives (and you learn quickly there is no such thing as an ordinary family!). Part of my training involved observing families like the one above without interacting with them. Family observation meant being a fly on the wall while families ate meals, debated who was taking the bins out, and argued. It became clear after a while that children in families absorb countless hours of interaction templates for everything; from showing love, disgust, and competitiveness, to the appropriateness of showing pride, laughing at outsiders, and imagining a future-self becoming a police officer or a career criminal. Family observation convinces me to draw connections from the client's experience of being familied to their current interpersonal patterns and ways of experiencing the world. Most counselling models have noticed that the experience of childhood influences the psychological and social trajectory of people, and the systemic approach pushes this further to consider all transitional points when working as a counsellor. Not necessarily giving priority to childhood.

Problem Timelining

As a counsellor it becomes essential to unpack family lifecycles because people are not only unaware of the hidden forces of lifecycles, but they actively dismiss lifecycle explanations before they are given time and space to process them. As the counsellor, we focus on the timing of the problem and the relationships around the problem, asking the client to think about what function the problem is serving in relation to the people involved in the problem.

For instance, we draw the timeline of the problem with a watchful eye or ear on moments of transition in the client's life. Timeline (a) in Figure 4.1 shows a client with the presenting problem of being angry and controlling. Timeline (b) shows the presenting problem of low mood and (c) the problem of anxiety. Each of these timelines highlights a lifecycle that gave rise to a psychological problem, supporting the systemic orientation we are exploring. In the case of (c), the anxiety occurred at a time where the male was approaching the stage of life for making a commitment to his partner and she wanted to move in together. In the case of (b), the problem occurred at a time of divorce, and in the case of (a) the problem occurred when a new partner moved into the family home. Each person develops a psychological problem because they are non-consciously renegotiating a new relationship and are using anger, controlling behaviour, anxiety, and low mood, functionally, to stick to an older pattern of relating. To keep someone new out of the family home. To avoid moving into a new family home. Or to prevent the breakup of a family home.

Family counselling often involves multiple family members in the session because problematic interpersonal patterns are more visible in the room. The psychosystemic problems are shiftable with more perspectives to unravel, provided the counsellor can withstand the difference of opinions, clashes of perspectives, and selective memory that supports and denies the selective memory of others, creating feuds, battles, and arguments. Using the timeline involves mapping over time where the issue emerged and pausing to reflect on transitional experiences and to openly negotiate the rules,

Timeline (a) Anger

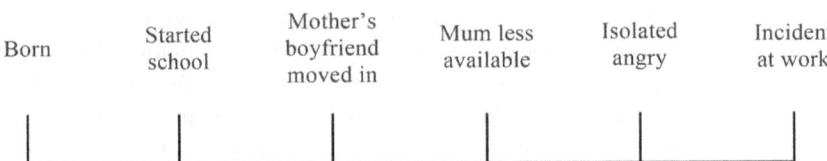

Timeline (b) Low mood

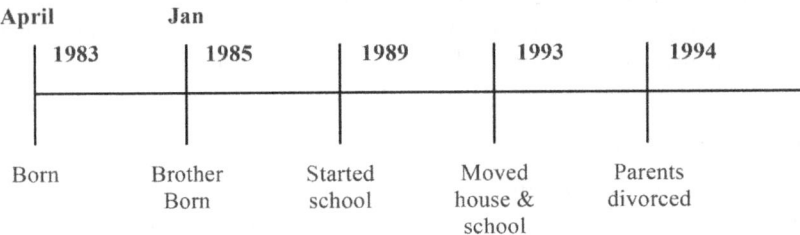

Timeline (c) Anxiety

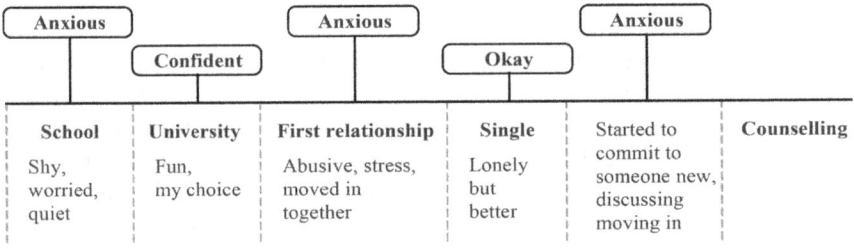

Figure 4.1 Problem Timelines: Timeline (a) Angry and Controlling Behaviour, Timeline (b) Low Mood Timeline, (c) Anxiety

boundaries, hopes, and desires of the new relationship. Often this involves some form of mourning the old relationship and life stage. We invite clients to think about what they need in the new stage of life in order to reduce the need for the problem.

Social Constructionism

We are going to talk in more detail about how to work with non-conscious rules and boundaries in the family system. And we will explore how family rules are formed, why they become outdated, and how psychological issues develop from lifecycles. First of all, we need to say a word or two about social constructionism to get to grips with an important implication from systems theory.

Language researchers have found that the meaning we place on an object, an event, or a relationship does not come from the object itself but from the people observing and discussing the object. For example, what does it mean to be a good mother? Well, by being mothered in our cultural setting, by seeing images of mothers in the media and television programmes, and by hearing people speak of "good mothers" and "bad mothers" we internalise the concept of a mother. Vivian Burr writes about this in terms of the theory of social constructionism, which means that values, beliefs, and meanings about things like mothers are socially constructed through social feedback and human interaction. Human systems are meaning systems. Through our habits and patterns of interacting, we construct images of other people and link their actions to our moral system. I should also say that anti-postmodernists claim that authors such as Vivian Burr are saying that "nothing really exists" and "all there is, is what we believe". And I think this is exactly wrong. It isn't that, say, the physical object of a good mother does not exist, but simply that "good" and "mother" are things people construct themselves rather than existing independently in the world.

In Chapter 2 we looked at reframing, where the meaning and definition of a relationship determined how a person experienced that relationship. Reframing is a form of social construction whereby something that once symbolised, say, fatherly authority in the transference relationship, now symbolised, say, care and compassion in the therapeutic relationship. Social constructionism happens at the linguistic level, in the words we use to describe ourselves, other people, and the environment, as well as at the active level, in terms of how shared action continually creates meaning. What meaning do you make of one person smiling at another? Well, it depends on the context. What is the relation between the two people? Is the smile happening in a supportive context or an oppressive context? A smile, like a mother, or a piece of music, requires a socially constructed context to be experienced as a good or bad thing.

Family Scripts

We develop ideas about ourselves, our lives, and relationships through social constructions in the form of stories and narratives. By story we don't mean something fictional or invented, but rather a way of making meaning out of the things we experience. Family scripts is an idea from developmental and cognitive psychology that an individual develops a script for what to do in certain circumstances, and these scripts contextualise interpersonal patterns. For instance, the circumstance of being a mother. Or the circumstance of being a son. Family scripts are the shared expectations of a family for how rules are supposed to be performed in a given context like a mother-son relationship.

There are hundreds of family scripts with layers of implicit rules. There are parenting scripts that contain lines about how to handle disagreements, express emotions, discipline children, show affection, encourage or discourage children from leaving home, and manage bereavements. There are gender scripts about family gender roles, traditions, beliefs, values, chores, housework, and caring. There are cultural scripts about the family's accepted or unaccepted identities, things to be proud of, things to be ashamed of, values around education and fashion, and social expectations. There are generational scripts about how different generations do the caring for one another, acceptable alcohol use, violence, displays of affection, ideas about what is right or wrong. There are problem-solving and conflict-resolution scripts, responding to anger, who takes control, democracy, and authority.

Family scripts are acted and re-enacted through interpersonal patterns. When a child is given a fire truck or a cute doll for their birthday, they are positioned to act within the boundaries of a gender script. When they react by accepting that position, the family praises them and showers them with affection. When the child reacts by going off-script, like a booing audience, the family automatically provides negative feedback loops. Sometimes of a harmless kind: "Oh he is special and likes to play with girly things". Other times in more coercive and damaging ways.

Using the family scripts approach, a counsellor turns away from lifecycle transitions towards beliefs and values. Circular questions draw out the interpersonal loops, and the family scripts approach is a way of explaining and making sense of those loops. For instance, the counsellor notices that a client hides his emotions from important women in his life, such as his ex-wife, his mother, and his boss. The client is asked about his family scripts in these contexts. What are your values around showing your emotions as a son? Perhaps he says that a son "should" always be respectful. Or perhaps he says that sons "should" never show aggression to their mothers. These "shoulds" imply rules internalised by repeated enactments of a family script. Drawing out the "shoulds" and the scripts in a client's life allows the counsellor to question the circular effects of the pre-written rulebook. Where did this rule develop in your life? What parts of the rule work for you and your mother/boss/ex-wife? What parts of the rule hinder you? Is this the ideal rule or would another rule suit you more at this time?

The psychologist who developed the idea of family scripts, whose name is John Byng-Hall, found that scripts can be altered when clients learn to improvise how they respond and react to others. He noticed that the most common scripts were linked with family experiences. People inherit scripts in such a way that they appear in one person and reappear in a descendant of that person. There are scripts that are repeated from generation to generation or from society to individual, and these are called replicative scripts. Then there are scripts that correct and challenge family and social scripts, and these are called corrective scripts. Usually, corrective scripts attempt to correct some negative, oppressive, or unhelpful script, such as a person who will never drink alcohol because their parent was an alcoholic, or a person who would never raise their voice at their children because they were repeatedly shouted at as a child. The third type of script is the improvised script or innovative script, which gives a client the autonomy to write a new script within a given context. Improvisation can happen when old solutions don't work, out of curiosity or fun, or when it feels safe to try something new. Often this is the goal of family counselling, to re-write scripts that prevent family development and impede individual wellbeing.

The Genogram

Family scripts are written and re-written in the performance-like interactions between family members. The structure of a family, which includes family relationships, family hierarchies, and family roles, is mapped out using the family tree or family genogram. Unpacking the family structure brings together the work on lifecycles and family scripts because they explain why the family is organised in the way it is.

To explore the family genogram, let's look at a referral that was made after a mum (Sharon) had found my number online following concerns about her son's (Nathan) cannabis use. She had found a small cannabis bag hidden inside his school jacket and found him occasionally to be high on weed. She asked if somebody could work with them as a family to stop him from continuing to smoke, which had been significantly affecting his schoolwork. Nathan's anger was a cause for concern, and he was beginning to be withdrawn at home when challenged about his cannabis use.

The family tree or genogram is a systemic tool that maps out the members of a family and the quality of their relationships. We start by taking a large piece of paper, ideally A3 size, and drawing one person on the page. To select the person, we ask the client(s) to decide who to draw first and the client's reasons for choosing them. Using the key in Figure 4.2, we identify the gender of that person. Why the gender? Well, there seems to be no real answer to this question other than that's the tradition in family therapy. Feminist and transgender activism has allowed for a diversity of gender expressions on the genogram and this allows multiple gender expressions rather than pigeonholing people into a binary view of gender.

Now you have found the symbol and drawn it onto the map, you have some important choices. Who next? For simplicity, I recommend drawing either the partner(s), sibling(s), or parent(s) of that person next. Let's say our client is Nathan and he draws himself first. Then he decides to draw his brother and their two parents. How do we represent this? Well, we use straight lines that lead from the top of the client's symbol to different levels, like different floors of a building. People on the same level or floor are from the same generation. So, children and parents are separated by one floor and children and grandparents are separated by two floors (Figure 4.3).

Once the family is mapped out, we draw lines between family members. Parallel lines indicate strong bonds and parallel squiggly lines indicate conflicted relationships (Figure 4.4).

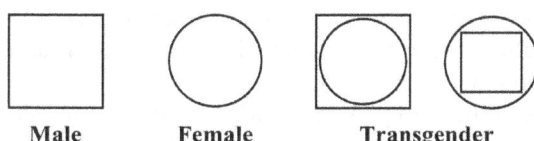

Male   **Female**   **Transgender**

Figure 4.2 Gender on the Genogram

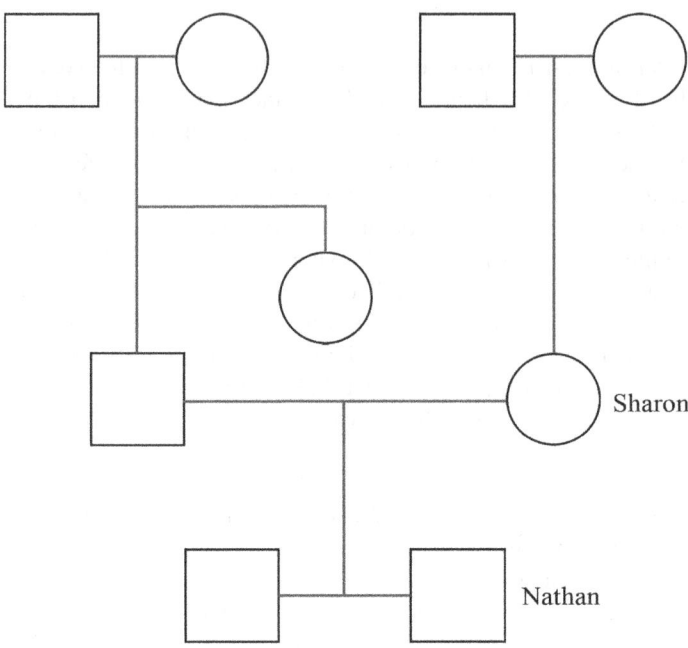

Figure 4.3 Levels of a Genogram

In my work I often use genograms with young people and their families to create a kind of cultural framework that adds unique meaning to their interactions. I use the Hardy and Laszloffy method of the Cultural Genogram. This is about having both awareness and sensitivity to the family's culture. Firstly, Nathan's family defined their cultural origin as White British, and we organised the elements of their culture into pride and shame issues. They identified that in their family being competitive, academic, and aspirational are all proud attributes, while being free-spirited, lazy, and unsuccessful are shameful. We then created the symbols that defined different cultural aspects, such as naming who is defined as aspirational and who is defined as free-spirited, and then identified connections between individuals within the system (Figure 4.5).

Triangulation

We can use the genogram to explore relationships between people and parts of the family system. We connect the quality of relationships with the issues of pride and shame, and these tend to reveal important family structures.

Nathan describes himself as one of the family members who is a free spirit. The family agrees that his mum and his brother are more academic and driven. This has created a coalition between Jack and Sharon against Nathan. Minuchin calls

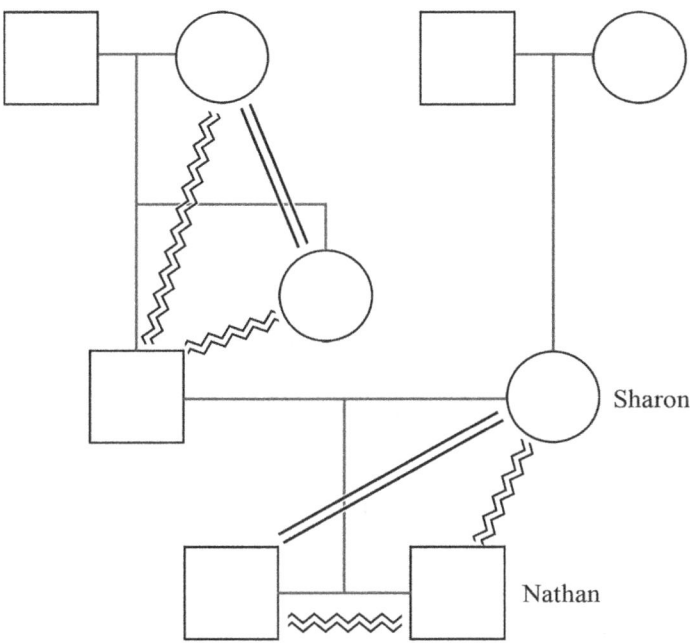

Figure 4.4 Relationships on a Genogram

this the rigid triangle, which is a situation when family values push members into different ideological camps. If Nathan acts free-spirited and stays in bed until 10 am, his brother notifies mum who wakes him up. If Jack acts driven and academic, Nathan mocks him for being conformist and brainwashed. Jack tells mum. And when mum complains to Nathan that he is not keeping up with his schoolwork or tidying his room, Jack sticks up for her. In these interaction patterns, the three become triangulated.

The observations from Murray Bowen show that families tend to develop triangulation, counterintuitively, as a way of stabilising the family. If mum becomes too driven for Nathan, then Nathan advocates living in the moment. If Nathan advocates living in the moment, Jack studies harder. The more the people change their position the less they change their overall pattern. What is stable is the relationship, even if the triangulated parties end up with psychological problems. Sometimes children's behaviour stabilises the parents. For example, conditions like anorexia force parents to overcome their relationship problems to prioritise their child's health. Sometimes conflict between one child and one parent stabilises the role of the golden child. For instance, the child develops a personality that serves the function of being a bad example. The most common triangle is the angel-and-devil child dynamic in families. People often don't realise how each role shapes each other role.

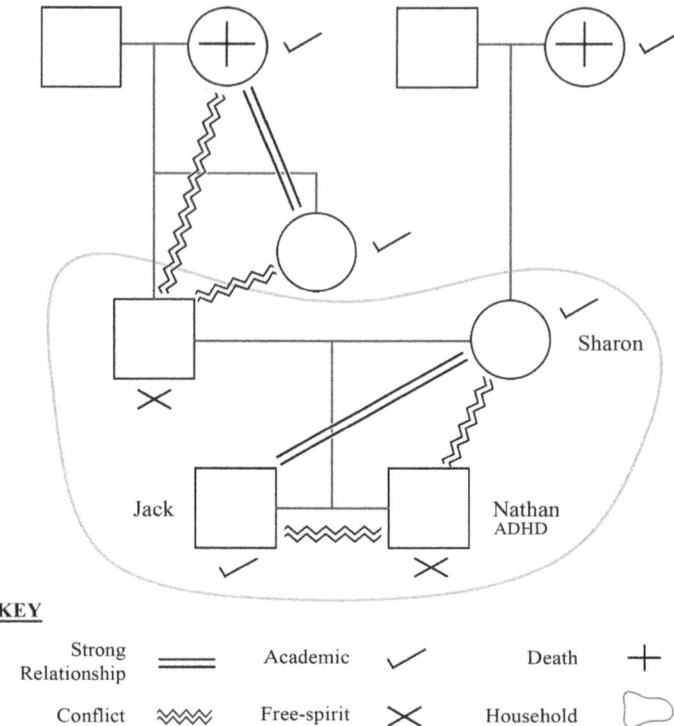

KEY

Strong Relationship	═══	Academic	✓	Death	+
Conflict	〰〰	Free-spirit	✕	Household	⌐⌐

Figure 4.5 Cultural Genogram

It is important to work on triads when seeing clients. Triangulation often repeats throughout generations. Nathan's genogram shows that triangulation had in fact occurred between his father, uncle, and grandma. The stability is often with the cultural value. That is, if the family changed their values, the triangles would dissolve or would shape around different family coalitions. The way a lifecycle comes in is that Nathan, being the oldest child, through his very existence brought a couple into a parental system, which activated a replicated family script around being academic. The script not working for them, perhaps because the parents struggled to attend to his needs while they negotiated the transition into parenthood, perhaps because he brought some learning difficulties with him that challenged the usefulness of the script, or for other reasons, the patterns between mother, father, and son become entangled by social expectations that fall out of their family values. A second child is then born four years later, and Nathan serves as an example of what not to become. His problems in the counselling room are linked with his family history.

Hypothesising

The family's history influences the types of patterns that family members create with each other, some of which make individuals psychologically unwell. In systemic counselling we attempt to describe the patterns rather than give an ultimate explanation for the patterns, mostly because valid perspectives on why the patterns happen are endless. Drawing on the famous work of the Milan team, who developed many of the current training approaches to systemic psychotherapy, we explain the pattern by creating a self-aware hypothesis. And an explanation that can change over time. Systemic hypothesising means connecting the lifecycle, family structure or scripts, and the family's interpersonal patterns into a circular description of the presenting problem.

Hypothesising is inspired by the work of Gregory Bateson. He said some important things on the idea of taking multiple perspectives on client issues, using the analogy of vision. Bateson discussed that seeing in three dimensions is possible because a person takes in visual information with one eye and combines it with a second eye to add depth to what they are seeing. Bateson discussed how the counsellor's metaphorical eye on the situation can combine with other eyes to create more depth from a multiplicity of perceptions. For example, seeing anxiety as an individual characteristic is like shutting one eye and saying that the world is flat. You flatten it with the way you look at it! So too do we flatten the client's problem by seeing it as stuck inside them. Double vision or, in the language of systems theory, double description is a way to add depth to a person's vision on their social reality. The problem with linear thinking is that all individual descriptions like anxiety collapse a three-dimensional reality into a single dimension.

In drawing the genogram, we become curious about how family members tell their story. Which realities are they evoking? What types of events, relationships, and problems do they describe? What does this say about their perspective?

The parents' story is that Nathan is a child with attention-deficit/hyperactivity disorder (ADHD) using drugs to look cool and fail his exams, which has led to stealing, appreciation of aggressive music, and hopelessness. In Nathan's view, he was liberated from the ADHD label by his friends who helped him to reduce stress by the introduction of cannabis, from which he has found his "only passion in life" as he aspires to a career in the music business: he sees himself as basking in hope "full" ness. But whichever way they conceptualise the problem, the family all agree that life together is stressful and at breaking point.

My systemic hypothesis was that Nathan's learning difficulties were seen through the lens of an academic family script, leading his academic mother and brother to form a coalition to attempt to increase his drive and ambition. Nathan's response to the coalition was to defend against it, becoming anti-academic and developing an anarchistic identity around cannabis culture, and this strengthened the coalition between mum and brother. Dad remained distant because he too was labelled as the undriven one in his family, and in not choosing sides between mum and Nathan he ends up absent from the discussion, giving the triangulation more room to thrive.

Hypotheses are not fixed formulations but evolving and changing ideas about the systemic issue. The Milan team famously warned against "marrying your hypothesis" because it can impose itself on clients indirectly through questions and techniques. There are three common shortcuts to hypothesising that stem from a value for multiple perspectives:

1. Structural: problems are maintained by the family organisation or family structure, the invisible or covert rules that govern the family's transactional patterns
2. Strategic: the problem serves a function in the family; if counsellors work on the function the problem is not needed
3. Lifecycle: the problem is because the family is being asked to reorganise relationships based on biological and cultural transitions

One example of a secondary hypothesis comes from strategic family therapy, whereby a problem is considered to have an important interpersonal function. Nathan's parents appeared distant, in the sense that they always sat apart and never touched or expressed a marital bond, but also in the sense that they appeared to talk through and around, rather than with each other. The strategic hypothesis was that Nathan's problems brought his parents closer together and distracted them from their own relationship. The reason I do not explore this idea in the session is that I feel it caused me to read their behaviour in the same way they read Nathan's, as stemming from disorder and failure. But creating multiple hypotheses is important before and after seeing families or individual clients, to ensure our ideas do not become forms of power and oppression. We are not in the business of trying to teach families the reasons why they have issues, but to create ideas that fit with them enough to undermine the problem.

A structural hypothesis would be that dad's absence leads mum and Jack to become a pseudo-parental system, responding to the concerns in Nathan, but having the effect of Nathan feeling ganged up on and retreating to a problematic peer group. If mum and dad are supported to communicate and co-parent, then the siblings could have a better chance of getting along, with the effect being that Nathan accepts and adheres to more of the family values.

The Circumplex Model

Circular hypotheses can be linked to the circumplex model, which provides ways for understanding family functioning. Family interactions can be dynamic and complex, and the circumplex model breaks these interactions down into three simple components: flexibility, cohesion, and communication (see Figure 4.6).

Though the circumplex model seems overwhelming at first sight, once a counsellor unpacks the different sections it can be used effectively for creating systemic

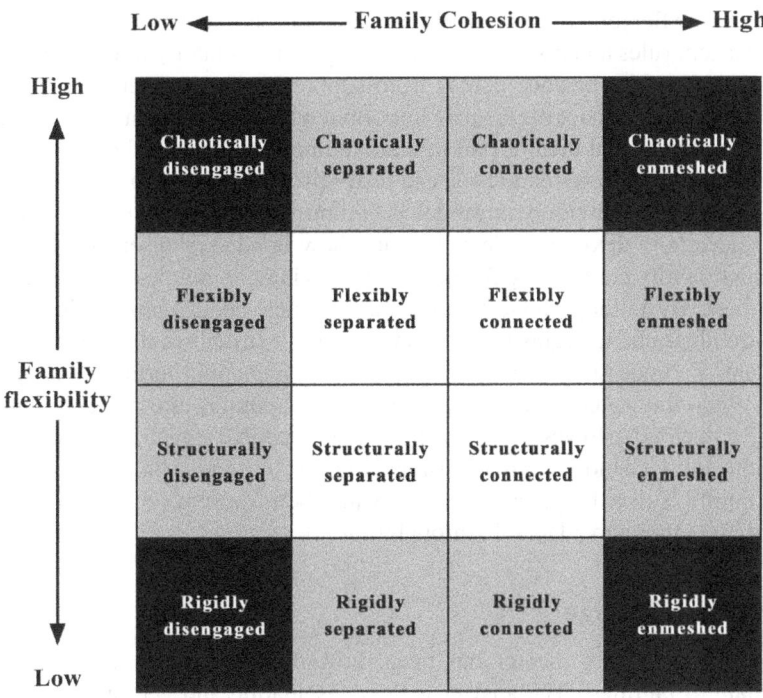

Figure 4.6 Circumplex Model

hypotheses and for knowing which areas to work on with families and individuals. The model encourages counsellors and families to strive for balance in their cohesion, flexibility, and communication.

Cohesion is described as the level of emotional bonding, including how connected and in tune family members are with one another. If the family members talk from a position of "I", have little closeness, loyalty, or dependence, then they are said to be disengaged and non-cohesive. On the flipside, if family members only speak as a "we", have extreme closeness, loyalty, and dependency, they are described as enmeshed. In situations like this, the goal would be to support the family to tolerate separation while staying connected, keeping a balance between these two extremes.

Flexibility is linked with how the family changes its roles, its leadership, and its rules. Being too rigid and authoritarian, where roles are fixed and rules cannot be explored, will stick families in time and prevent their development across the life-cycles. For instance, a common example is a child who begins school and develops an anxiety problem because the change in role of being a school child, of being more independent, cannot be tolerated by the parent-child subsystem. A child may cry and show distress. Or a parent may overly worry and ask frequent questions about the dangers of being in school. The other extreme can also be problematic. On the other side of the flexibility spectrum is chaos, where chaos means a lack of leadership, inconsistent rules and discipline, creating big shifts in family roles. In terms of flexibility, the healthy balance comes from supporting family members to be flexible yet structured. It is not necessarily important which family member you see as a counsellor; each one of them is part of maintaining the system and counselling support for anyone, with a systemic lens, can prove useful in changing the system.

The final part of the circumplex model is communication. How people communicate decides how flexible or rigid they are, how bonded or disengaged they are, and as such family counselling focuses on improving communication between family members. By talking about bonding, about rules, about family roles, the family or individual client begins to work on the family structures that contribute to the problem. To understand the circumplex model, one could form an analogy with water. When the water is heated up, the water evaporates into a chaotic and unstructured gas cloud. However, when the water is cooled down and frozen it transforms into solid ice blocks. An enmeshed family is like an ice block whereas a disengaged family is like the gaseous state of water; both cause problems in keeping the family together and adaptable through time.

The Process of Change

The basic question of this chapter has been, how do individual psychological problems relate to families? The answer is very fascinating and yet very simple. Problems occur mostly with the birth of a child, during adolescence, launching, and so on, because these moments are transitional moments where families must re-negotiate the unquestioned (and safe) structures of their relationships. Because relationships are held together by rules that are unspoken and unconscious, this negotiation tends to happen via behavioural responses and emotional disturbances. McGoldrick called these "life cycles" because cultural and natural transitions force families to rewrite the important codes of conduct that previously held sanity in place.

When families hold rigidly to their current rules, such as that parents monitor children every hour or that partners spend time together every evening, feedback escalates and escalates until change occurs or the system becomes strained, something Minuchin termed a "transitional crisis". With Nathan's family we brought out family stories that contextualised his mother's framing, such as the idea that when children do poorly in school, they are lazy or unaspirational. His mother was enacting the cultural story that being a good mother means helping children become educated, and these stories were born out of social values and beliefs. For Nathan, who had in mind a different family script, his mother was in the category of a "bad mother", because his script was around being free-spirited. These scripts developed to spite one another, to make sense of conflictual, triangulated family dynamics.

Families grow and change through time to meet the developing and changing needs of their members. The external and internal demands for change are continuous but become critical at transitional points in the family's life. Problems arise from attempted solutions, whereby a solution attempts to keep people inappropriately in an old pattern of relating. Such families need to make changes at these critical transition points, such as changing the family structure, beliefs, or emotional dynamics.

The Internalised Genogram

With individuals, drawing a genogram can be exciting and useful. There are also times where it is time-consuming and stale because the client does not know how others experience the family system. The internalised genogram is a shorter but effective technique I developed for counsellors who want to work with family dynamics but more quickly and with individual clients. The client is asked to draw the members of their family, as they see fit, on the page. Once completed, the familiar process of adding symbols, words, and connection lines applies. Usually how clients represent their family dramatically expresses their internal, felt experience of being part of the family system. This is also permission to think outside the traditions of genograms and to use them in ways that meet client demands. Many counsellors don't use techniques that feel overly complex and simplifying them is better than avoiding them.

In one example of the simplified genogram, the client was asked to draw their family on a blank page. They drew themselves and their mum on one side of the page, and their step-father and step-siblings, much bigger, on the other side of the page. In drawing relationship lines and symbols they began to articulate an experience they had been holding onto, that their family was split in two. The action of drawing was part of the unravelling of the meaning and experience of the client. They had been puzzled as to why they could not get along with their step-father, and visualising the family interpreted this for them. In being a split family, their hostility towards their step-father was supportive of their mother. His children had not accepted being part of the household since their biological mother was in the picture. Here we found a family script, a lifecycle change, an interpersonal pattern, and a triangulation, simply from having the client draw their family, getting rid of the need to use the formal symbols.

In my experience, teaching and drawing genograms is problematic because the skill and memory-power needed to organise a complex family into a neat structure is astronomical. The internalised genogram is a reminder that the practices in counselling are open to interpretation and change. An example comes to mind of an internalised genogram drawn by a child in an adoptive family, in which their drawing signified that everyone in the family was happy but them. They drew a tangled line from their hand to their adoptive sister's hands to represent being hurt by her. Towards the end of the family counselling, after some months, the child re-drew their genogram and showed a marked difference in their internalised sibling relationship. In this second drawing, she and her sister had vibrant smiles and were sensibly linking hands without discomfort. The child was not languaging the felt change in relationship, but, in freeing ourselves from the structure of the traditional genogram, we were able to feel what it was like to be inside the old and new relationship artistically.

Further Reading

Bachler, E., Frühmann, A., Bachler, H., Aas, B., Strunk, G., & Nickel, M. (2016). Differential effects of the working alliance in family therapeutic home-based treatment of multi-problem families. *Journal of Family Therapy, 38*, 120–148. doi:10.1111/1467-6427.12063.

Bowen, M. (1985). *Family therapy in clinical practice*. Lanham, MD: Rowman and Littlefield.

Burr, V. (2015). *Social constructionism* (3rd ed.). London: Routledge.

Byng-Hall, J. (1985). The family script: A useful bridge between theory and practice. *Journal of Family Therapy, 7*(3), 301–305.

Carter, B., & McGoldrick, M. (Eds.). (1988). *The changing family life cycle: A framework for family therapy* (2nd ed.). New York: Gardner Press.

Haley, J., & Richeport-Haley, M. (2003). *The art of strategic therapy*. New York: Routledge.

Minuchin, S. (2012). Families and Family Therapy (2nd ed.). London: Routledge. https://doi.org/10.4324/9780203111673.

Olson, D. H. (1993). Circumplex model of marital and family systems: Assessing family functioning. In F. Walsh (Ed.), *Normal family processes* (pp. 104–137). New York: The Guilford Press.

Rosen, K. H., Lechtenberg, M. M., & Stith, S. M. (2015). Strategic family therapy. In J. L. Wetchler & L. L. Hecker (Eds.), *An introduction to marriage and family therapy* (pp. 155–181). New York: Routledge.

Selvini, M. P., Boscolo, L., Cecchin, G., & Prata, G. (1980). Hypothesising – circularity – neutrality: Three guidelines for the conductor of the session. *Family Process, 19*(3), 12. https://doi.org/10.1111/j.1545-5300.1980.00003.x.

Chapter 5

Contextual Behavioural Counselling

In the previous chapters, we discussed that psychological problems arise from repeated behavioural exchanges described as interpersonal patterns. Buried beneath this simple idea are two complex and mutually reinforcing concepts that have profoundly shaped the direction of counselling and psychology over the last 100 years. The first is to do with the theory of behaviour and the second with the question of how people make meaning from behaviour. In this chapter we explore the rise of cognitive and behavioural concepts in counselling and integrate them with systems theory.

Behaviourism

To integrate systemic ideas into the contemporary world we must visit the renowned theory of behaviourism and, following on from behaviourism, examine the fruits of the cognitive revolution. Part of this book's aim is to reject the prejudice in some counselling and psychotherapy writings that different models of therapy are incompatible, when usually they are different ways of explaining the same thing or are simply paying attention to different aspects of the client's problem.

Behaviourism brought a fresh perspective to the interactional model of human wellbeing by studying how interactions between individuals and their environment mutually shape and reinforce behaviour. In its basic form, behaviourism is a theory that claims that people and animals become conditioned into patterns of reflexes or behaviours when paired with specific stimuli. All behaviours are learned from the environment and the more positive reinforcement for a behaviour the more likely it is to occur.

Conditioning

Conditioning is the foundation of behaviourism and is the label for a process of associating behaviour with positive or negative feedback. Overcoming a mental health problem according to behaviourism requires individuals to change their reactions to situations by learning new responses. People are rewarded or punished for different behaviours and become conditioned into behaviours that avoid

DOI: 10.4324/9781003480808-6

punishment and seek reward. There is a link here between psychodynamic theory and behaviourism because, in both models, individuals are understood as driven by a pleasure principle, but the argument from the behaviourists is that their theory discusses only scientifically measurable things like behaviour. Unobservable things like unconscious drives and internal states do not feature in a behaviourist's description of counselling, only the fact that through reward and punishment people become conditioned into stereotyped behaviour.

Behaviourism shows that if a person is punished for showing emotions, for example, they become conditioned into behaviours like withdrawing or denying feelings when an emotional topic comes up. As the withdrawing behaviour is reinforced, that is, when someone is mocked or frowned at for showing emotions, by a parent, a partner, or a sibling, the negative feedback increases the likelihood of withdrawing behaviour. Counselling re-conditions people's responses to relevant stimuli using positive reinforcement from the counsellor. For example, a counselling client who becomes withdrawn (response) when discussing emotions (condition) might learn to cry, show anger, or express anxiety when the counsellor persists in asking questions about emotions, providing them with positive reinforcement when they discuss feelings.

Graded Exposure

Graded exposure is a form of conditioning that gradually reinforces desired behaviours with a client, slowly and supportively exposing them to a trigger situation, and is a powerful example of how to alter a person's behaviour linked with that trigger, usually with the effect of reducing any associated emotional distress.

An example springs to mind of working with a teenager in a school for young people with trauma backgrounds. Rio was 15 and came to an alternative education centre where the policy was to undergo a mental health screening by me as the school therapist, attached to a local authority mental health service. The centre wrote her referral form and highlighted disruptive behaviour, truancy, low mood, anger, and her conflicted "attitude" towards her mother. Rio was first introduced into a routine therapy group with six other young people. She refused to talk about herself and displayed frustration towards my inquiries, saying that counselling was "rubbish", and that she hated her previous counsellor. She sat out of the group activities and appeared low in mood while the other young people joined in. I observed that Rio rarely interacted with peers and her lack of engagement disrupted others who stopped the activities to engage with her throughout the session. Rio was invited to meet with me the following week for a mental health assessment. She refused.

Habituation

In behaviourist terms, inviting Rio into therapy was a stimulus for her refusals and frustrated behaviour. The school had noticed a pattern of her refusing and withdrawing from activities, particularly when the situation or event was labelled as being supportive to her, emotionally. Behaviourism uses the concept of habituation to explain how people with repeated stimulation of a behaviour form a relatively permanent set of responses to specific situations: they become habituated.

Over the course of a few weeks, the school and I shifted the plan of counselling to the plan of graded exposure to attending counselling so that the automatic response of "refusal", "withdrawal", "frustration" could be altered in a positive direction. The freedom for an integrative way of working is to use these ideas with the system around the client, particularly if working with clients in schools or mental health hospitals where offering counselling becomes caught up with stimuli around authority and histories of abuse. To re-habituate the client we need not have them in the room but can plan the intervention in such a way that gradually exposes the client to therapeutic and trusting relationships.

Hierarchy of Exposure

Grading the exposure from low to high, smallest to biggest, or least difficult to most difficult, is a common way to work with clients in figuring out how to support them from a set of habituated responses to more-favoured altered responses (see Table 5.1). Since Rio was refusing to attend counselling, the staff team and I discussed ways to gradually include her in counselling conversations.

The behaviourist method demonstrated that counselling was the highest possible trigger for Rio. Thinking in terms of graded exposure allowed us to rethink ways to reduce triggering stimuli by slow and thoughtful contact with me as the school therapist.

We decided that I would sit with Rio in the social area during the lunch break where students sat around and talked informally (lowest trigger). The next week I opted to play games with her and her peers (low trigger), and she was particularly competitive with a card game called UNO, which was safer and less triggering (and enjoyable!). Eventually, Rio began to trust me and agreed to attend the mental health assessment, fairly quickly, once we had established a relationship. Graded exposure can dramatically change phobic behaviour to behaviour that is relaxed and comfortable in previously distressing environments. With Rio this was a useful way to conceptualise change, as an intervention of counterconditioning.

Table 5.1 Graded Exposure

Trigger	Rank (High to Low)
Counselling	Highest
Group counselling	High
"Normal" lesson	Medium
School outing	Low
Social time games	Quite low
Lunch time	Lowest

A Systemic View of Behaviourism

Behaviourism is the factual account of a systemic worldview. That is, behaviourism has studied countless interpersonal patterns and shown that they shape individual behaviour and wellbeing. A systemic orientation can integrate findings from behaviourism by using meaning-making tools to help clients and therapists make sense of the context for things like habituation against counselling.

Pride and Shame Stories

When we eventually convened the mental health assessment, Rio presented with a tense relationship to the kind of help that focuses on her mental health. In our first session, we constructed her genogram (Figure 5.1) where she noted cultural values around gender, that girls are helpers and boys are doers, and she discussed how she had grown up with her father and older brother (the doers) but with restricted contact with her mother, sister, and youngest brother. At the start of counselling, she had not seen her mother for around six months.

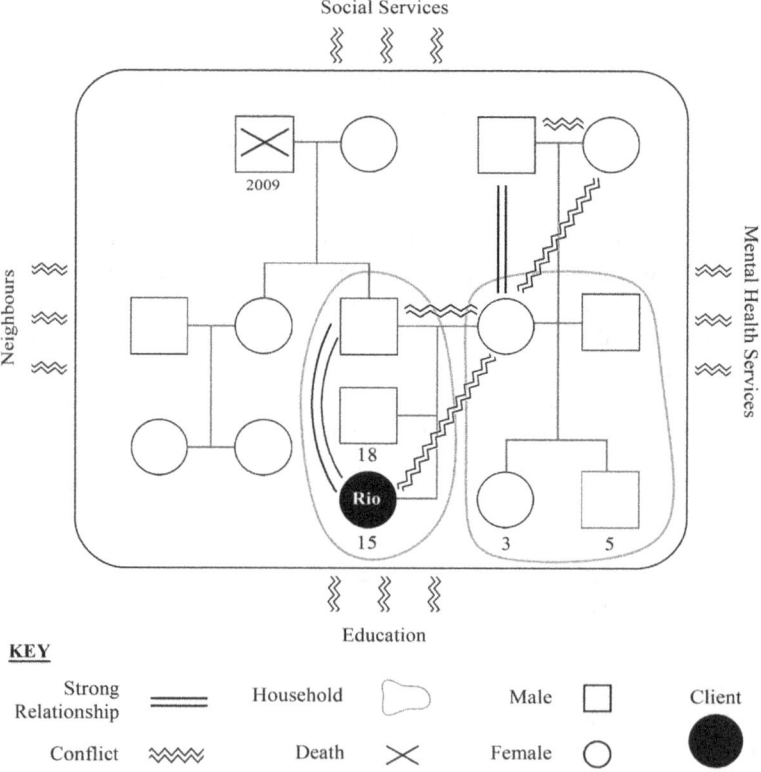

Figure 5.1 Genogram and Ecomap

Hardy and Laszloffy discuss the importance of counsellors identifying areas of pride and shame in family stories, and this was helpful for Rio because she connected talking with issues of shame in that she experienced blame, shame, and manipulation when seeking emotional help from her mother but supportiveness, care, and comfort when seeking practical help from her father. In behaviourist language, Rio has been reinforced into being pragmatic and against having or showing emotions. In systemic language, this issue has created an alliance between Rio and her father against her mother, which, in Chapter 4, we referred to Minuchin who calls this the rigid triangle. Bowen studied how triangulation often repeats throughout generations and Rio's genogram shows that triangulation occurred between her mother Mary and her maternal grandparents (Figure 5.1). The two triangles are repeated, with both females being in a coalition with their fathers against their "hateful" mothers. This family tree activity was useful in Rio understanding her opposition to my help as a counsellor and undid some of the resistance to it, particularly when she realised that she has nowhere in which her emotions and vulnerabilities can be openly expressed.

Isomorphism

In systems theory, isomorphism is when a group of people like a family replicate patterns that are symmetrical with other groups like a school. Usually, interaction patterns are replicated from one system above or below another system in a social hierarchy. For instance, Rio has a gendered view of problem-solving and this influenced an isomorphic pattern to develop from her family situation into her school community. At age 13 she experienced trauma from a series of serious bullying incidents and was referred to school counselling. Her view was that counselling, which invited her into emotional help with a female therapist, was frustrating and unhelpful. She decided that in order to feel calmer she needed to avoid seeing the bullies—a practical male idea—but the school was said to disagree, and the bullies remained in the same class while Rio was encouraged to resolve her difficulties in counselling. For Rio, the school's approach fragmented her relationships with teachers and strengthened her view that emotional help can be blaming, something she learned from her mother relationship. This is isomorphism because the school culture was replicating the family culture; they were similar in structure and the structure was related to how mum and teachers responded to Rio not wanting emotional types of support. Rio felt that the school system constructed her needs as emotional, and the problem then became a seesawing effect between her and school. The more Rio showed a need for practical help, the more the school viewed her as in need of emotional help. As professionals we often replicate the split in families by being against one parent, or both parents, so children and parents form coalitions against us, which was true in this case as dad did not originally support counselling in her mainstream school and agreed that the bullying was the only problem. Rio's recollection was that she solved this problem by truanting and being disruptive, for which the school permanently excluded her.

In Rio's case, behaviourism does not need the baggage of context or a case history to help her through therapy, but in doing so loses the richness of a systemic lens that supported Rio to make meaning out of and have more control over how she does or does not seek support. Moving between a practical behaviourist approach and a family tree activity seemed to create something more than the sum of the two approaches. And it was an attempt to step out of the stuck position, which we have discussed as isomorphism, where the school began to replicate the family triangle in which Rio was in the middle of two contradictory values: practical help and emotional help. It is possible too that Rio's alliance to her father influenced her rejection of motherly-feeling-type responses to her needs.

Cognitive-Behavioural Therapy

The claims of behaviourism have been tested by rigorous scientific methods. Most famously, the Russian psychologist Pavlov showed that laboratory dogs are conditioned to salivate on hearing a dinner bell as though the bell itself was the same as the smell or sight of food. That is, behaviour in the form of salivating, crying, and refusing therapy has been shaped and changed experimentally by offering different conditions to the human or animal. When environmental conditioning happens, the behaviour of the individual becomes habituated for better or worse in terms of their wellbeing.

The cognitive revolution challenged behaviourism to think about its underlying structure. What is at the root of behaviour? Why have we neglected experiences like thoughts or feelings? What is the relationship between the way someone thinks and their behaviour? The answers to questions such as these transformed modern counselling and psychotherapy practices and evolved into the most researched and discussed form of psychotherapy of the 21st century: cognitive-behavioural therapy, or CBT.

Where the cognitive revolution challenged behaviourism was to suggest that much of what people think and feel, internally, motivates or explains their behaviour. Later these theories would combine into the contemporary use of cognitive-behavioural therapy pioneered by Aaron T. Beck, who showed experimentally that thoughts, emotions, body sensations, and behaviour are connected. What we think and do affects the way we feel in circular ways. Removing this cognitive chain from the description of behaviour was seen as simplifying and muddying important aspects of psychological problems. Researchers such as Fordham et al. have reviewed the evidence and concluded that adding the cognitive focus to behavioural therapy led to counselling techniques that dramatically reduced individual problems like depression and anxiety.

Formulation

CBT expands on behaviourism by saying that behaviour and indeed mental health, anxiety, depression, and emotional distress are maintained through cycles of unhelpful cognitions and maladaptive behaviours. A case formulation, which is a hypothesis about the presenting problem, from a cognitive-behavioural perspective, highlights how a problem has a set of psychological mechanisms and other factors that are causing and maintaining it.

CBT uses this general or so-called nomothetic formulation for every counselling client, in that thoughts, feelings, and behaviours maintain presenting issues. It goes further to say that specific or idiographic formulations can be made with each client where clients map out cognitive-behavioural cycles, the mapping-out being a form of psychoeducation and insight into the problem. This then allows CBT-informed counsellors to work on coping strategies, challenging unhelpful thoughts and behaviours, repeating and reinforcing new behaviours, and preparing for relapses.

The Hot Cross Bun Model

The most notable way of turning a general formulation into a specific, idiographic formulation is by using the Hot Cross Bun Model, named for its physical resemblance to the white cross on the top of a hot cross bun. This technique visually represents the cognitive-behavioural theory, recalling this to mean that thoughts, feelings, and behaviours mutually influence one another in repeated and often-escalating cycles.

Figure 5.2 is what was described earlier as a nomothetic formulation, in that it generalises all mental health problems into cognitive-behavioural boxes. Through the use of the various arrows, it depicts how cognitive and behavioural dimensions intersect. When the client fills out this worksheet, whether by drawing it as shown or by answering carefully constructed questions from the counsellor, who might

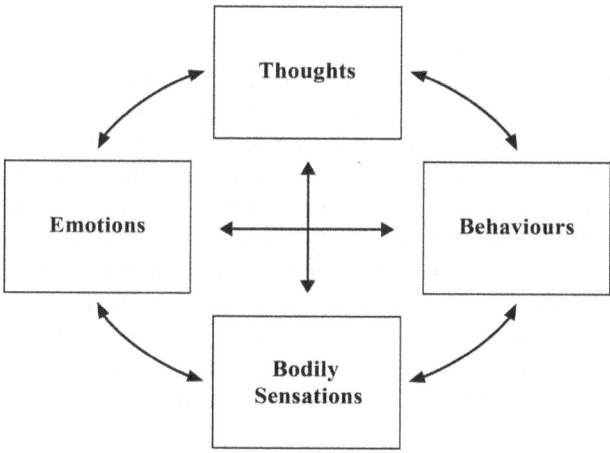

Figure 5.2 The Hot Cross Bun Model

imagine filling out the worksheet as they question the client, it becomes an idiographic formulation, one that is specific to that client. So, Rio thinks "counselling is rubbish", feels "frustrated", and responds behaviourally by "refusing therapy". This was a move away from behaviourism in psychology, a turning towards what has come to be known as the cognitive revolution, shifting intellectually to a position of seeing behaviour as the result of internal mental and cognitive processes.

One of the intellectual giants of behaviourism, BF Skinner, said that all behaviour is unconscious but becomes conscious when one analyses it. In this idea he collapsed the need for a Freudian unconscious in psychotherapy and promoted the idea that people gain insight and reinforcement by looking at their behaviour, an early form of psychoeducation. If a client like Rio could gain insight into her cognitive-behavioural cycles, then she could reinforce thoughts and behaviours that overcome her emotional difficulties. In this sense, a CBT formulation is a form of intervention because understanding the problem as cognitive-behavioural cycles changes how the client experiences their issues.

Systemic CBT

The way a systemic psychotherapist would move forward with this idea is to study the behaviour as part of a sequence rather than only the outcome of a conditioned response. The integration of a systemic approach draws attention to the context for the cognitive-behavioural cycles. In fact, Beck's original cognitive theory was based on observations that people with depression tended to hold negative views of themselves, the world, and the future. This negative triad, as he called it, stemmed from depressed people's implicit and core beliefs about themselves, such as believing they will always be unhappy, or that the future has no purpose. In this way, CBT views context first as a set of core beliefs and second as a way of experiencing situations, and this was diagrammed in Padesky's first hot cross bun model (Figure 5.3).

Gregory Bateson challenged the work of Pavlov and the other behaviourists by showing with humans and animals that conditioning doesn't happen with a stimulus but a stimulus in a specific context. One example is with orcas (killer whales) whereby the whale learns to associate food rewards with flapping its fins to a hand gesture or squirting out water at the blow of a whistle. When the whistle or hand gesture was given outside the context of the swimming pool, the whale did not have the same behavioural response. In effect, a person or animal creates meaning from an event such as a hand gesture within a specific situation. Changing the situation changes the meaning of the hand gesture and the behaviour because behaviour is a response to a meaning someone creates in a given situation. An interesting finding from this experiment was that when the whistle or hand gesture was unclear, the whales began to show disturbed and psychotic behaviour … More on this in the next chapter.

A useful clinical example was given by a client dealing with anger difficulties. Something interesting happened that day that really consumed her thinking. In the

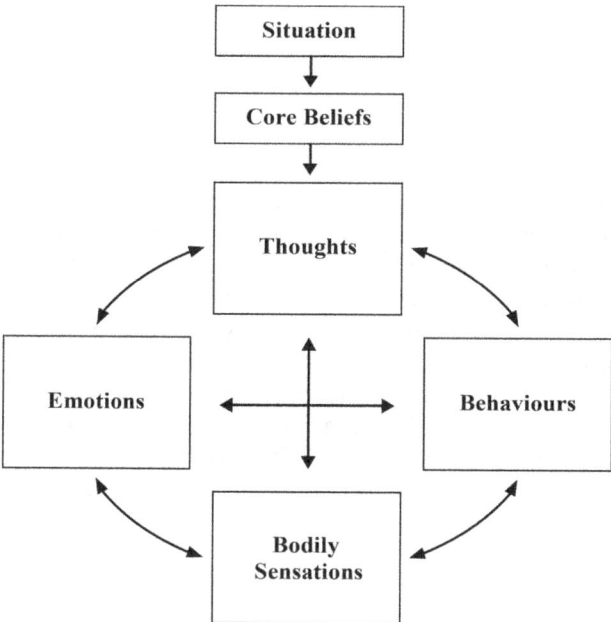

Figure 5.3 Padesky's Hot Cross Bun Model

morning someone she fancied was repeatedly sending her messages on her phone. Each time the sound rang she said she felt a rush of excitement and described the sound, in her words, as like "cocaine". Yet, a few hours later, her mother kept "going on" at her with a barrage of text messages about a family feud and suddenly the same notification sound—the same stimulus—became a source of great irritation, to the point of her becoming furious and smashing her phone against her computer desk. The same notification sound was dramatically transformed in a matter of hours due to a shift in context. It was stimulus plus context that set the stage for the excitement and the anger responses, and crucially this led to opposite behaviours.

Connected with this, an experimenter named Konorski replicated the famous Pavlovian experiments but sneakily removed the sound of the bell without the experimenter knowing. The dog still salivated! The conclusion therefore was that the dog, instead of being conditioned by sound alone, was conditioned by context instigated by the sound of the bell, the sight of the bell, and presumably the friendly human bringing the dog a set of curious items. Bateson's and Konorski's research does not undermine the earlier findings of the behaviourists but shows us that the layers of conditioning are complex. In fact, Konorski was the neurophysiologist who coined the term "neural plasticity" because his experiments indicated that the brain must wire and rewire itself to different environmental input within certain contexts, a process he defined as learning.

A Reminder of Context

Context is a frame for how someone understands and interprets a situation, object, or relationship. The metaphor used in systemic therapy is not to condition people to behave differently but to learn new contexts for experiencing. This is encapsulated well by the metaphor of "reframing" that we met in a previous chapter, and reframing counselling for Rio was achieved via the route of graded exposure. Systems theory draws attention to the inevitability of behaviour change when a client reframes their lives. Bateson would say that Rio has learned a contextual structure, a set of rules for how to put the information together in the school or counselling context and we can use cognitive-behavioural cycles to help clients like Rio to question and challenge the rules they implicitly live by. Padesky's hot cross bun model suggests that situations are experienced through learned beliefs, and this is consistent with the systemic view of context.

Putting the Thought on Trial

One way of contextualising cognitive-behavioural cycles is the activity known as "Putting the Thought on Trial". Because CBT has specialised in cognitive thinking, it has developed a wide vocabulary to describe types of thoughts that create problems for clients, as shown in Table 5.2.

Table 5.2 CBT Categories of Thought

Type of Thought	Definition
Arbitrary inference	The client draws conclusions without appropriate evidence.
Selective abstraction	The client focuses on one negative aspect of a situation and ignores more favourable aspects.
Overgeneralisation	The client applies one narrow conclusion to a broad range of situations, often based on one-off situations.
Magnification/minimisation	The client enlarges or reduces the importance of events and discounts the positives.
Personalising	The client relates external events to themselves and inappropriately sees things as personal.
Catastrophising	The client assumes the worst possible outcome and overestimates the possibility of it happening.
Mind reading	The client assumes awareness of what others negatively think or feel about them.

The most common way to run this activity encourages the client to take negative thoughts that are relevant to the problem and act like a courtroom, cross-examining each thought. CBT counsellors refer to this as cognitive restructuring because to put each thought on trial is for the client to restructure their way of thinking about the thought and implicitly to restructure their way of thinking about themselves, the world, and their future, having the potential to change their future behaviour. Rio could put her thought "counselling is rubbish" on trial and we might ask what the evidence for this thought is and what the evidence against it is.

Thought: Counselling Is Rubbish

Evidence for: I had a bad experience with counselling and felt blamed for my problems. I find talking about problems difficult.

Evidence against: The counselling I have at the minute feels helpful. Counselling seems to work for some of my friends. I think it's good to talk to people when you're feeling upset or annoyed even if it is difficult.

At the end of the activity, each thought is then given a verdict by the client, such as whether the client-as-judge rules the thought to be true or untrue, helpful or unhelpful, and we might work with the client to modify the thought. Thought modification simply means having the client rewrite the thought in language and, like a chant, to practise using this thought when in need of a positive perspective. The thought is put on trial by examining evidence for and against the thought and the client judges the thought, often in a playful way, to be guilty or not guilty of contributing to the presenting problem.

Scaling the Thought

CBT encourages counsellors to scale the thought across different contexts or situations, to support the client to unpack the contextual structure of their thought. Thus, integrating the CBT technique with systems theory is made possible by asking the client how their thoughts change in different relationships and systems.

The technique is to take the thought and place it into different environments. Rio's thought "It's hard to talk about problems" can be met with the question: "in what situations is it hardest to talk about your problems?" and "in what situations is it easiest to talk about your problems?". The situations can be ranked and ordered in such a way where the client creates a context-dependent scale of the problem. For example, Rio might produce something like Table 5.3:

The counsellor now has information about five different contexts that are important to the functioning of the problem. They can begin to unpack the context by asking about "why" or "how" it is easier or harder in different situations, supporting the client to uncover the implicit rules they follow within a given situation.

Table 5.3 Scaling the Thought

Situation/Person	Rank
Mum	Very difficult
School	Difficult
Counsellor	Quite difficult
Dad	Okay
Friends	Easy

A Reminder of Feedback Loops

From what we have said so far, how is the client seen as benefiting from the reframing and unpacking of the contexts or rules that overlook their experience?

Systems theory is formulated on the assumption that people's actions maintain patterns (or relationships) that keep them in balance with each other and their environments. A famous yet obscure quote from Parsons (whom we met in Chapter 2), "action is system", means that one cannot do an action without interaction. Much of psychology has focused on the action or the behaviour of one individual without having noticed that the individual's action takes place in relation to other actions. With this in mind, how do people keep cycles of interaction going, non-stop?

A key figure in systems theory is Norbert Wiener, who, having worked on anti-aircraft guns during the First World War, showed that shooting down enemy planes required an understanding of the relationship between the movement of the plane and the gun handler. As the plane moved through the sky, bombing the towns and cities below, the gun handler needed to use the plane's position as feedback, in order to change his position for a more accurate shot. Wiener showed that feedback was a way of controlling a system by reinserting into it the results of its past performance. The plane, in avoiding the gunfire, would see the spraying bullets too as feedback, adjusting its direction and position accordingly. A context of war was the basis for systems theory, which, as we said in Chapter 3, was referred to as cybernetics, and which showed that systems keep their balance by using continuous feedback loops. Behaviourism uses the concept of feedback as a linear process without commenting on the loops and cycles that maintain systems.

The thermostat metaphor became the central way of understanding feedback loops. Hot and cold temperatures tell the radiator what to do in the context of a thermostat setting. I had a funny experience of this at the Tavistock Clinic where I did my early training, because the thermostat for the air-conditioning unit was placed directly next to the window, meaning that when the window was open the feedback to the thermostat was breezier than the room actually was, so the air-conditioning would not work. A paradoxical situation happened every summer where we had to close all the windows in a hot room in order to cool it down.

Similarly, Bateson and other system theorists found that people keep their balance through feedback loops within a social context, and often they behave in seemingly bizarre or paradoxical ways like refusing counselling when they need someone to talk to.

Theory of Learning

Returning to Rio and her problem of finding it difficult to talk about problems, we can now apply the concept of feedback to her situation. Wiener showed in systems theory that recording or "taping" (like the old cassette tapes; taping the radio for example) occurred whereby people record, save, and remember ways for interpreting information from a special perspective. When people change the taping or method for how they interpret events then this is called learning. The systemic theory of learning is that through joint action people create and maintain interaction patterns that maintain their stability (their homeostasis). When the method for interpreting events is changed then these patterns are also changed, and systemic learning has occurred. John Burnham calls this a change in the definition of the relationship, and we have named this a second-order change.

When Rio thinks it is harder to talk about problems with her mother than with her father, there is an implicit context that she responds to in the climate of her respective family homes. Rio behaves differently in the presence of her friends than her schoolteachers not because she has a faulty cognitive structure but because her cognitive-behavioural cycles depend on the context in which they take place, on the interpretive frame of that context. Learning about the frame or definition of the context takes the person outside of their assumptions about the only possible realities within a system, relationship, or environment. The relationship between Rio and mum may always remain set in stone. But Rio's way of interpreting emotional help can develop.

The physiological basis for second-order change is well established. Functional magnetic resonance imaging (FMRI) scans have revealed that brain cells link together in new formations to generate new ways of perceiving the world. This neuroplasticity, in which the brain rewires itself to the environment, means that people can recover from trauma, overcome bad habits, and acquire tastes and preferences for new experiences. Change requires people to de-couple things like emotional help from rejection or blame, and learn to associate emotional help with things like care and compassion.

Contextual Behaviour Therapy

An important advance in understanding Rio occurred by integrating cognitive-behaviourism and systems theory. The thought "it's hard to talk about problems" is strong enough for a person to avoid counselling. But how does systems theory account for this thought?

In families, the emotional balance is always struck between its members. It is therefore economical to dissuade some emotions when other emotions would be overwhelmed if allowed out. A parent who cannot contain frustration at a crying infant will feed back frustration when the child cries. Such a response from the parent may have to resist the infant's cries initially, but after that, the child cries less and less not because they are feeling cared for, but because the pain experienced from the parent's frustration develops in them a conditioned reflex that prevents the child from outwardly showing their needs. In this situation, the original trigger to the reflex is fear or pain. The sight of the parent then becomes a trigger or a context for withholding needs when they arise. As the child grows, they transfer this learning onto other caregivers or contexts in which needs arise in them. Through different caregiving environments the child learns a variety of contexts for displaying emotions, as well as the feedback from how others display emotions and the types of responses given. Systems theory would wonder about the parent's way of being parented, for example, and avoid linear explanations, which tend to end up in mother-blaming despite the context being that mostly mothers, and even more so mothers who have themselves been abused, are deemed responsible over fathers and society for rearing children in under-resourced and isolated situations.

As a child like Rio grows up and her brain develops to think, feel, and somewhat take ownership of her behaviour, she expresses her system of relationships through refusing counselling and being excluded from school. I completed some research with young people like Rio and found out that most excluded children are understood through the lens of behaviour problems when living in abusive or socially deprived contexts that lead to behaviour problems. Our feedback to clients like Rio is part of creating a context for changing the way she perceives care, or for restructuring her cognitions, as CBT languages it, against the background of family and community difficulties. Putting her thoughts on trial or teaching her about the hot cross bun model of psychology is attempting to create a new context for how she perceives herself. People are not machines in that the memory is embodied and not simply recorded in digital form, but the principle that people remember associations and patterns to determine how they behave in the present moment is hugely supported in the research.

Recall that earlier phrase from Wiener, that feedback controls a system by reinserting into it the results of its past performance? With Rio we are helping her to see that her past performance of help-seeking has controlled the way she seeks help. By unpacking the contexts through techniques like scaling we can learn more about how she wants to respond to support. When feedback or information is used to create successful changes with clients, Bateson refers to this as "a difference that makes a difference".

Systems theory adds to behaviourists like Pavlov, Skinner, and Beck the notion that behaviour is coordinated together. The environment is conditioned by the individual and the individual by the environment. We can develop a contextual behaviour counselling approach by asking clients how other people respond, what other people feel, what other people think, to their cognitive-behaviour cycles, helping clients learn about interpersonal patterns and cognitive processes.

The counselling plan was to help Rio fit in more with peers and lower her frustration. There was no conscious intention for her to build bridges with her mother. But after a while Rio came into the session and announced that she had been to see her mother, spontaneously, and they had a much-needed chat. Rio did become more comfortable in school, and we had a counselling relationship right until her last day of school. Reflecting on my experience of working with her, I think switching between a frame of thoughts-feelings-behaviours and a frame of systems and relationships was important. Rio didn't thank me for the work done, despite building up to the point of using me as her "agony aunt" every week, something I very much valued. But when the time came to end counselling, she did say I was not the worst therapist in the world and that seeing me wasn't all bad.

Further Reading

Bateson, G. (1980). *Mind and nature. A necessary unity*. New York: Bantam Books.

Beck, A. T. (1993). Cognitive therapy: Past, present, and future. *Journal of Consulting and Clinical Psychology*, *61*(2), 194–198. doi:10.1037/0022-006X.61.2.194.

Fordham, B., Sugavanam, T., Edwards, K., Stallard, P., Howard, R., Das Nair, R., … Lamb, S. (2021). The evidence for cognitive behavioural therapy in any condition, population or context: A meta-review of systematic reviews and panoramic meta-analysis. *Psychological Medicine*, *51*(1), 21–29. doi:10.1017/S0033291720005292.

Greenberger, D., & Padesky, C. (1995). *Mind over mood: Changing how you feel by changing the way you think*. New York: The Guilford Press.

Hardy, K. V., & Laszloffy, T. A. (1995). The cultural genogram: Key to training culturally competent family therapists. *The Journal of Marital & Family Therapy*, *21*(3), 227–237.

Konorski, J. (1967). *Integrative activity of the brain*. Chicago: University of Chicago Press.

Murphy, R. (2022). How children make sense of their permanent exclusion: A thematic analysis from semi-structured interviews. *Emotional and Behavioural Difficulties*, *27*(1), 43–57. doi:10.1080/13632752.2021.2012962.

Parsons, T. (1978). *Action theory and the human condition*. New York: Free Press.

Pavlov, I. P. (1927). *Conditioned reflexes: An investigation of the physiological activity of the cerebral cortex*. Oxford: Oxford University Press.

Skinner, B. F. (1988). *About behaviourism*. New York: Random House.

Chapter 6

Communication Counselling

The most common feature of psychotherapy is the use of language or the "talking cure", yet most counselling models have no theory of language, no theory of communication, and no theory of meaning. How strange it is that the very thing that expresses the pain and suffering of the client and the careful attention of the counsellor is invisible to the books and papers of most psychotherapy authors. It is like being an expert in boating with no concept of water. In this chapter we present a systemic theory of communication alongside a variety of systemic techniques that have been developed for counselling individual clients.

In the late 1900s, systemic ideas met with social constructionist ideas. Each set of ideas explained two parts of the same observation. The social constructionists saw that people came to know the world around them by creating perspectives or social constructions. Language was shown not only to describe but to shape reality. On the other hand, the systems theorists showed that nature, humanity, and society remain in balance by feedback loops, joint action, co-evolution, circularity, communication, and group relationships. Language and communication systems are the media by which societies assemble and are the water in which social relations remain afloat. The merging of social constructionism and systems theory led to a focus on communication, language, and meaning as the basis for problems in counselling. In this chapter, we probe into the communication theories that sprang from this time. We explore ideas about language and social discourse in the next two chapters.

Communication Theory

The theory of communication was introduced by the mathematician and engineer Claude Shannon. He defined communication as any process where one mind affects another. Leaving this theory extremely broad, Shannon explained how communication works through body language, music, writing, aggression, and, of course, language. His main preoccupation was with computer communication, yet the foundation of his work was general systems theory, or GST, which we mentioned in Chapter 1.

DOI: 10.4324/9781003480808-7

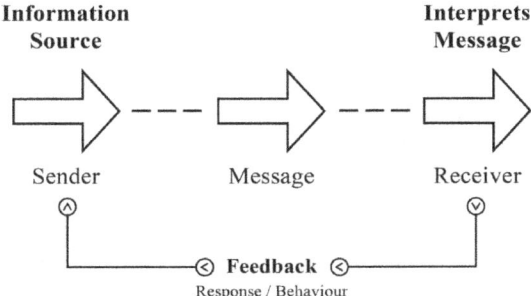

| Information | | Interprets |
| Source | | Message |

Sender   Message   Receiver

Feedback

Response / Behaviour

Figure 6.1 Shannon's Communication Theory

Shannon showed that communication involves at least three levels (see Figure 6.1). Level 1 is the technical level for how accurately symbols are transmitted from one location to another. Level 2 is the semantic level for how accurately the meaning of the symbols is conveyed. Level 3 is the effectiveness level for how well the received meaning affects the behaviour of the receiver of the signal.

A quick study of these levels shows how these three simple ideas apply to all communicational systems. A dog barks (Level 1). A would-be intruder interprets the bark as "I will bite you" (Level 2). The intruder runs away (Level 3). A counsellor nods head (Level 1). A client interprets the head-nod as "I care about what you are saying" (Level 2). The client opens up emotionally (Level 3).

The bark of the dog, like the nodding head of the empathic counsellor, is a symbol for care or aggression that is transmitted through sound (barking) and sight (nodding) to the receiver, affecting them in some way. Communication takes place when one mind, dog or human, affects another.

Inaccuracy of Communication

Communication theory highlights that not all communicators and receivers are 100% accurate. Sending and receiving messages through words and behaviours, inherently, causes some static or background noise. A problem develops whereby if 10% of the communication signal is wrong, it cannot be that 90% of the message is transmitted because the receiver may not know which parts of the signal are wrong. For instance, let's imagine a child takes the anxious yet exciting first movement to crawl away from a parent (see Figure 6.2). When the child turns, they're frightened about the distance from their parent. The child seeks reassurance from the parent, to assess the level of risk, by smiling or frowning. If the communication works, the parent smiles or frowns back depending on how safe the crawling is perceived to be by the parent. A distracted parent, perhaps someone reading a newspaper or making lunch, will have shown an unreadable face. Perhaps the parent frowned and smiled at the same moment, creating ambiguity in their communication signal. This worries the child, and they begin to cry (the child communicates

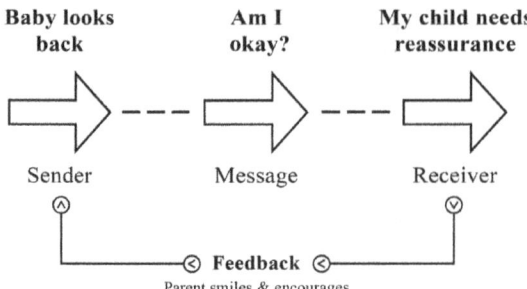

Figure 6.2 Communication Theory Example

distress) at this ambiguous communication, which draws in more proximity and reassurance from the parent. Instead of crying, an adventurous child might smile a second time to gain clarity over the signal from the parent. Asking the question, what does your face mean? This time, concentrating on the child's activities, the parent returns a beaming smile and encourages the child to crawl further, using affirming voice tones. Though crawling is a cognitive and physical developmental milestone, the child learns to crawl through communication and feedback loops. Ambiguity is normal, and people and animals take enormous strides to work out and correct inaccurate communication signals. The good news for parents is that securely attached children and their parents only attune about 30% of the time.

In communication counselling, the therapist is an observer, which Shannon rather unfeelingly refers to as an "auxiliary device". This is someone who helps clients process and understand the communications in their family and social systems, to work out the ambiguities, to reflect on the meaning of different communications, and to change how they communicate with and feed back to others (see Figure 6.3).

In the example from Figure 6.3, the client's partner is quiet. This source of information carries the potential message "I need space", but is picked up by the receiver, the client, and translated as "He is angry with me". In this communication system, what would be the client's feedback? How would this feedback affect their interpersonal patterns? Notice that an observer comes in, observing the source of communication, the message, and the interpretation. The counsellor-as-observer asks questions in such a way that corrects or changes the data from the partner, and the client reinterprets the message. Here communication theory is demonstrating how the feedback loop would change and possibly resolve the tension in the system.

The Stop Sign Activity

Communication theory seeks to unpack interactions using Shannon's three-level approach. This works well with couples and families, particularly as the system is

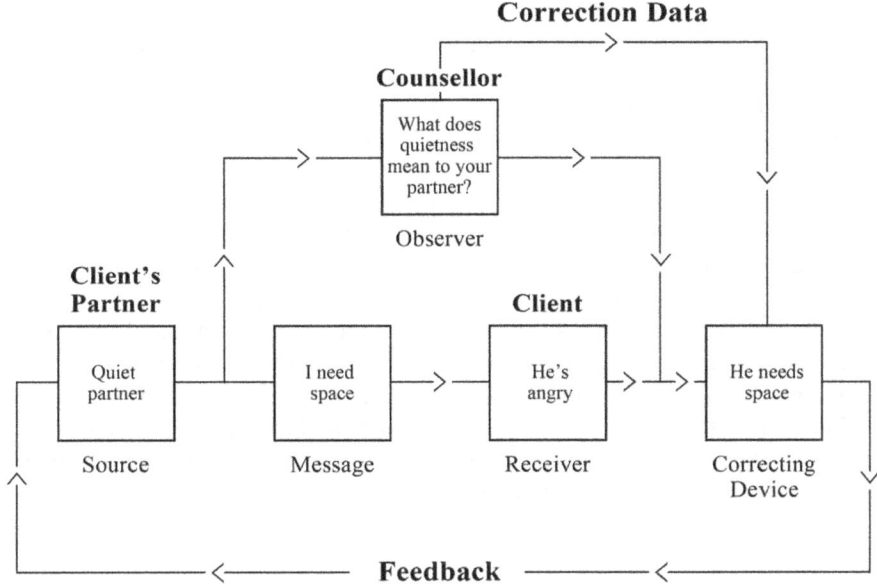

Figure 6.3 An Observing System

in the room with the counsellor. The adapted version for individual clients is also very effective and is called The Stop Sign activity.

In this activity, the client works on an interaction they found to be important to their presenting problem. Usually this is a distressing situation or an argument but could be a positive change or a dialogue that shows growth. The counsellor suggests that the client draws, writes, or explains the three levels as follows:

Level 1: Repeat and summarise what the person said or did (source)
Level 2: Consider, how did you interpret and experience what the person said or did? (receiver)
Level 3: Then consider, how did you respond, what did you do? (feedback)

A client gave the following example:

1: My work colleague messaged the group about having worked hard that day
2: I felt angry and upset and interpreted that they were saying that I was not working hard
3: I ignored the message and stayed later than usual to show that I am a hard worker

The client processes the difference between the message sent, the interpretation and experience, and the effect their interpretation had on them. It is possible to run through multiple rounds of the three-level dialogue. I would recommend doing this in real time with couples and families, asking each person, before they respond intuitively, to repeat what the person said or did, explain how they interpreted and experienced the communication, and then to respond. Many issues in counselling boil down to how the interpretation of the signal or communication is tangled into the signal or communication itself. The effect of this activity on my client was that she immediately realised she had created the competitiveness she felt in work instead of supporting her colleague with a message of gratitude. This was important for her because the reason for counselling was a feeling of social isolation despite being around and seemingly accepted by many people.

Communication theorists see that when a client hears or sees a signal from their environment, what reaches their sense organs seems different according to their perceptions. If a client lacks the perception and training necessary for seeing the possibility of being connected to others, this information will meet a block. The source information, what people said towards or did around them, would meet an interpreting structure that contributes to their mental health issues.

The Double-Bind Theory

A communications theory of mental health was put forward by Bowen and Bateson at different times in the 1950s and 1970s when studying schizophrenia and other chronic conditions. Using ideas from Shannon and other communication theorists, they noticed how psychosis develops in one person within their family communication system. The observations of families were very profound and shifted teams of psychiatrists from a diagnostic view in favour of a systemic theory of mental health.

The schizophrenia studies with families showed a very interesting thing. Schizophrenic families, as they were referred to in the studies, displayed high ambiguity in communication signals. Shannon had already shown that communication happens at the level of the word and simultaneously at the level of the voice tone. A contradiction between what is communicated, e.g. the words, and how they are communicated, e.g. the tones and gestures, makes the communication ambiguous for the receiver of the message. The term Bateson and colleagues used for the tone of voice and bodily gestures is "metacommunication" because it is a communication about the communication. Metacommunication is a higher form of communication that says something like "though I am saying the words 'I am fine', I am showing tonally and behaviourally that I am not fine". Bateson showed that when a person communicated love and metacommunicated something more like hatred, the receiver of the message, usually a child in a family, had no way of understanding or grasping reality. And this is incredibly important for the communication theory of mental health. It takes a moment to think outside of the ordinary descriptions.

To understand how reality gets lost in communication, imagine a scenario where you respond to the "I'm fine" words of your friend. Accepting the person is fine means they are likely to amplify their not-fine communications, perhaps becoming agitated, upset, or ignoring you. However, if you respond to the "I'm-not-fine" communication in the same tone of voice, you will likely be met harshly with a frustrated communication like "look, I said I'm fine, now you're annoying me!". In the same way as our schizophrenic families, if the child responds to the love communication they are met with a similar fate. The parent's hostility increases. But if the parent's hatred or disdain was responded to, then, as with the friend who says they are fine, their experience is contradicted: "But why are you so angry at me, all I did was tell you I love you?".

Bateson called this the double-bind theory. A double bind is a situation where a person is damned if they do and damned if they don't. Many of us have had the experience of seeing someone looking down and asking them how they are, and having them respond with that phrase mentioned above ... "I'm fine". If we respond as if they are fine, we get ignored or moaned at for missing the fact that the person is not fine (or we leave them alone and feel guilty ... guilt is such an activating social emotion!). On the other hand, if we respond to the metacommunication, to the annoyed or sad voice, then, like the person who develops psychosis, we are denied our experience and told in more frustrated terms that they are fine, and it is us who has the "real" problem.

Much of behavioural and language-based communication is double-binding and contradictory. Most of us cope well with ambiguous communication and rely on it to hide painful feelings or socially unacceptable intentions. But if we live in an environment of chronic contradictory communication then we lose our grip on reality. In this sense, reality is that event, situation, or action which we perceive as existing in our social world. This implies we need social confirmation to validate our reality. Schizophrenia was theorised as developing when people are unable to accurately interpret social signals within a tense and often hateful family experience. Autism is another example where difficulty interpreting social signals creates a tremendous amount of anxiety. If social communication becomes clearer, there is no anxiety or delusion.

The Double Communication Activity

The double communication activity invites clients to unpack messages within their communication. The counsellor asks the client to re-enact communications that are important for the counselling problem. As the client says these communications out loud, they are encouraged to pay attention to the signal (the words) and the way in which the signal is carried (the voice tone and body language).

One example comes from a client who wanted to address feelings of rejection from his mother. He was asked to write and then speak statements that he would ideally like to convey to his mother. He wrote:

You make me feel unloved.
I want you to take my feelings seriously.
Why don't you ever call me or ask about my life?

Once written, the client spoke these words to the counsellor. Open questions drew attention to different characteristics of the communication.

The client and counsellor noticed he clenched his fists when saying he felt unloved, possibly sending the signal that he is angry. He sounded dismissive when he asked for his feelings to be taken seriously. The tone conveyed messages of anger and frustration and the counsellor showed curiosity towards how the mother tends to respond to anger and frustration. The client discovered something important. In imagining communicating with his mother, he created a situation in which asking for her to meet his needs became a process of creating withdrawal in his mother. A systemic self-fulfilling prophecy was imagined, and this was a helpful realisation.

The client came to therapy because he wanted to be more confident and emotionally present in his life. In reflecting on the content of his words and the process of conveying them, he became more aware of how his passive voice tone and argumentative posture were part of inviting rejecting responses from his mother. For him, rejection and the anticipation of rejection were the basis for his low confidence and emotional avoidance. The history of this interaction sequence is important to highlight. But the history exists in the present. Clients show their communication history by the ways they communicate in the present, even with imagination and roleplay.

One benefit from this approach is that clients regularly take steps to communicate differently with the imagined other, usually a parent. Other times the communication history is frozen solid. The client sees no hope in thawing out their relationship. But in these cases, the client tends to harness self-discovery beyond the imagined relationship into important encounters with friends, partners, and colleagues. Communication counselling works on presenting issues like confidence, anxiety, and emotional avoidance by clients realising the anxiety or confidence issue is a signal inside a relationship, rather than a fixed personal characteristic. We move from "being anxious" to "showing anxiety" and focus on the pattern.

The Co-ordinated Management of Meaning

A person's communicational history creates a storage of memories for how to interpret other people's words and actions. The physiology of memory is well established, and brain-imaging technology has shown that brain cells link together in new formations and form new ways of perceiving the world. Neuroplasticity, as we have discussed in previous chapters, allows the brain to rewire itself to the environment. To paraphrase Von Foerster: the moment we see something differently, something new is there.

So far in the chapter, we have discussed communication theory in general. The work of Barnett Pearce and Vernon Cronen took communication theory into the specific context of human society, away from the nuts and bolts of computers and machines. In human communication, Pearce and Cronen noticed that people interact with the environment to create social structures and culture. Their theory is called the Co-ordinated Management of Meaning, or "CMM" for short, because their basic principle of communication is that people create societies and traditions through action and communication. This fits well with the ecological systems theory we discussed in Chapter 1, in which Bronfenbrenner described society as layered, moving from the individual person, their family, their community, and on to their wider society. CMM focuses more on the communication and meaning that gets created within the layers of society. In what follows, we will think about co-ordination of meaning at the level of two individuals interacting, and afterwards we shall connect the two individuals with the wider social structures to see how CMM theory explains the one in relation to the other.

The Co-ordination Map

To understand social co-ordination, communication counsellors find a way of mapping out the interactions between two or more people. For instance, let's say we are counselling a 14-year-old who has developed anxiety linked with her best friend having recently begun to self-harm. The cutting became so bad that her friend was hospitalised, raising the client's anxiety significantly. A co-ordination approach supports the client to draw out relevant interaction sequences, perhaps like a comic strip, or by using language, and particularly sequences in which the anxiety emerges.

Using the co-ordination map (Figure 6.4), the young person reflected on interactions where anxiety was the outcome. First of all, she went to her friend's house and asked how her friend was doing. Then her friend responded with a dismissive tone, asking not to be hassled. Afterwards, the young person asked again how the friend was feeling and encouraged her to open up emotionally. The friend then shouted and demanded to have no further questions. The young person felt paralysed by anxiety.

The pattern between the two friends is what Bateson refers to as a complementary escalation. As one side does more of the questioning, the other side does more of the refusing. Each person then escalates their behaviour until communication breaks down. From a communication perspective, each person is attempting to co-ordinate with the other, but failing. But why are they failing to co-ordinate? We know from Bateson what the pattern is, but why is this pattern happening?

The Episode

CMM theory puts forward that co-ordination is problematic when two people come together from different social realities. Complementary escalation and mutual escalation occur when two people attempt to recruit one another into their social way of seeing things. CMM theory calls this "rhetorical eloquence" whereby communication is aimed at convincing another person to accept their reality. We can understand this by taking a closer look at what the communication counsellor does to support the client.

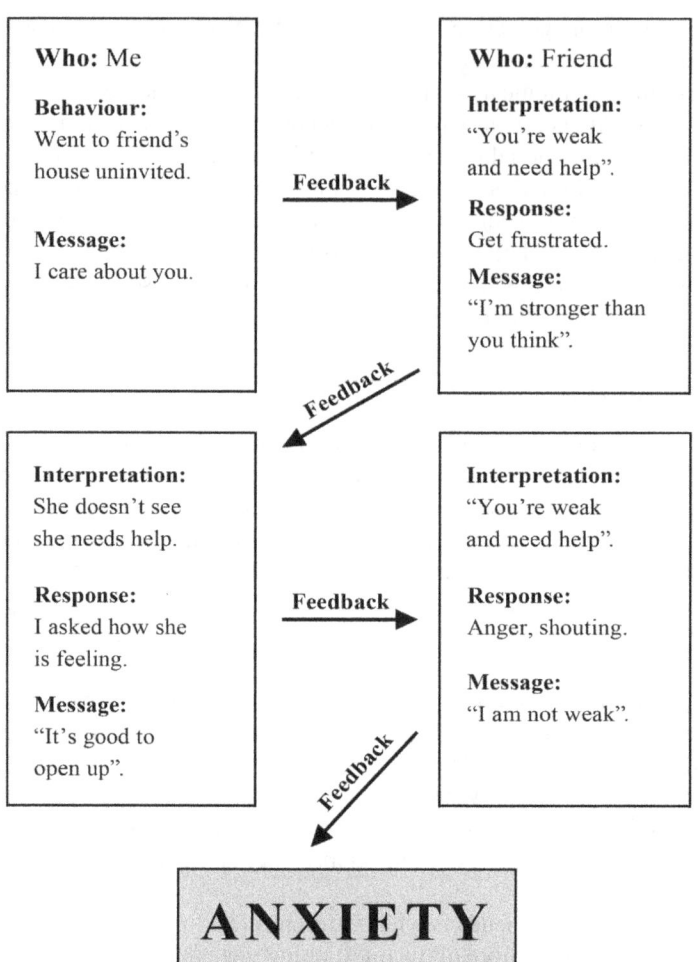

Figure 6.4 Coordination Map: Anxiety

The counsellor at each interaction point asks probing questions such as: Why did your friend behave like that? What were you hoping for from that move? How did she experience you when you asked questions? Asking questions about meanings brings the co-ordination map to another level; it helps the client move from rhetorical eloquence (or convincing) to "social eloquence" whereby the client is more able to co-ordinate their reality with their friend's reality. To understand this second level, which is the level of meaning-making in CMM, we need to briefly describe the CMM concept of "episode".

The concept comes from the starting point that common sense tells us that the world is clear to anyone who simply looks around. Pearce and Cronen challenged the common-sense view of the world to show that what we see is not a world that comes pre-packaged with meaning. We see a string of many happenings that through culture and experience we transform into a meaningful narrative. They said, "we cannot perceive all of what is going on even in a specific moment" and, to cope with this, we place events "within an interpretive frame" (Pearce, 2007, p. 137). In CMM theory this interpretive frame is called an episode. Think of an episode from a TV series. The episode is a frame that makes all the actions within the 20–30 minutes of happenings make sense.

Returning to the co-ordination map, the client can be asked to name the episode or reality that each person in the interaction is in. This allows the client to co-ordinate with the reality of her friend without giving up her own reality. Often mental health problems develop when two or more people compete to define reality. The client in question named her episode as "caring for my friend". She named her friend's episode as "hanging out". By naming the episode it was immediately clear that both people were attempting to bring the other into their own social perspective or episode, to use rhetorical eloquence.

Scripting the Episode

In drawing the co-ordination map, the client has made sense of her anxiety as the outcome of a communication sequence. She has then provided two ways of seeing this sequence, two episodes, which change the interpretation. This is the most important part of the activity. The client can now be asked to script the episode, something Pearce and Cronen referred to as doing "episode work", according to the two perspectives. In her perspective, she is attempting to care for a risky friend. By not accepting the friendly help to talk about her emotions, the friend shows more risk and even more need to be cared for. This explains the repeated questioning from the client and demonstrates a problem in the friend.

In episode two, "hanging out" or "I am strong", this second way of viewing the interaction shows that the friend wants to have a fun and relaxed time together and not be therapised. This frustrating pull towards the "you are weak" episode had been happening since she left hospital by almost every person she encountered. In the "hanging out" episode, the friend has legitimate cause to see the client as the problem. The more the client attempted to therapise her, the more she resisted and showed frustration.

Episode work is therefore an act of co-ordination. That is, it helps clients to move between different social worlds to gain systemic insight into the difficulties they encounter. The anxiety can be explained as a combination of systemic interactions and socially constructed interpretations that create escalation patterns.

Punctuation

CMM theory has shown that when two people produce an interaction pattern, they often describe the sequence of events differently from one another. It answers questions like: How is it that people come to experience events so differently? Is one person lying and the other being truthful? Is there some greater jigsaw puzzle of truth that each of them holds a piece of?

When people live in different or clashing episodes, they usually start the story of events in different ways. Pearce and Cronen refer to the process whereby events are organised in terms of a beginning and an end as acts of punctuation. For example, the "I care episode" begins with a traumatic hospital scene. The "hang out" episode begins with an annoying and patronising friend. These beginnings to each person's story significantly affect the meaning they make.

CMM explains how meaning is created from different perspectives about the most suitable way to punctuate a situation. For example, a young person presented at my clinic with the view that her mother's emotional withdrawal made her angry. The very next week we invited her mother in to help us to think about this; the mother reported to me that it was in fact her daughter's anger that caused her to emotionally withdraw. The mother and daughter punctuated the events very differently, and perhaps this was their problem!

When we unpack situations where there appears to be a continuous loop of events—such as the anger-creating-the-withdrawal loop—we find that the rules of interpretation change. A quick leap into the field of linguistics can help us to understand this phenomenon in more detail.

The journalist and grammarian Lynne Truss wrote an excellent book on grammar called *Eats, Shoots & Leaves* (try and spot the two meanings here). The book demonstrates how punctuation in sentences is responsible for creating meaning. For example, Truss gave the sentence below to prove that sentences can have two opposite meanings, simply by adjusting the punctuation:

A woman, without her man, is nothing.
Or
A woman: without her, man is nothing.

In this grammar exercise, Truss demonstrates how punctuating sentences in different places creates new meanings from the same string of words. In a similar sweep of the imagination, Barnett Pearce and Vernon Cronen noticed that human interaction is like linguistic grammar, or, more specifically, that human communication has its own grammar that produces different perspectives on events. Pearce and Cronen put forward that a circular interaction is paused or punctuated differently by communicators. The punctuation difference explains the difference in meaning.

Re-Punctuation

A communication counsellor can use the concept of punctuation to assist clients in overcoming individual problems. The technique is to have the client discuss an interaction sequence and, after the story has finished, support them to change the starting point, three or four times. This is because many people start stories with themselves as the respondent to a communication and as such take the victim or "done to" position, rendering themselves passive recipients of forceful communicators. Or they non-consciously edit their behaviour as the pseudo-beginning to the story, suggesting their actions as being agreeable to the outside observer. Clients run into problems when their ways of punctuating events chronically repress alternative edits of the sequence. In communication theory, all punctuations are valid but only some create exits from harmful interpersonal patterns.

In one example, a client told me that his sister had shouted at him for parking in the wrong car park en route to a family dinner. The client had constructed a reality in which he had made an honest mistake and the sister's rage seemed disproportionate. When re-punctuating the episode, the client said that right before the car park incident, he had not allowed his sister to drive because he "knew the best route". This new starting point to the story gave more merit to the sister's frustration. The client, in this punctuation, appeared to be naively controlling. In completing a further re-punctuation, the client said, just before offering to drive, that his sister was stressed in having to arrange a birthday cake—since they were travelling to their father's birthday dinner—and he had tried to show confidence in knowing the directions to alleviate his sister's stress. Suddenly he's a martyr!

The new punctuations generated a difference in how the client perceived the events. Many client problems are presented in ways that obscure aspects of alternative realities. We are ultimately trying to support clients to situate their experiences within relationships, circular causes, and interpersonal patterns, and in ways that co-ordinate between their social reality and others. In my experience, clients report that such trivial differences in how reality is perceived are experienced as significant in their mental health issues. The communication counselling approach places less importance on the content of the interaction, such as parking disputes or birthday parties, than on the process of communication and how interactions end in distress for clients.

People-Grammar and Homeostasis

The idea of punctuating the episode refers to dividing and organising sequences of interaction into meaningful patterns. The word "punctuate" and the word "divide" suggest that each episode is formed from a unique grammar that changes the meaning of the interactions according to how the dividing and punctuating is done.

CMM is more complex than at first sight. This is because the rules and the structure for how a person interprets or punctuates events are not random; they are socially made.

Let's briefly return to our analogy with grammar in language. The eminent linguist Noam Chomsky points out that the rules of grammar are usually not thought about by language speakers and if you ask the average non-linguist to describe how they know that English sentences are grammatically correct, they have no idea. Even the educated language student knows words like "verb", "noun", and "participle", but they usually cannot explain why English follows English rules in comparison to other languages that follow different rules. This unconscious system of grammar, of making meaning out of strings of words through punctuation, is analogous to the unconscious system of people-grammar, of making meaning out of strings of communication and interaction.

Like the unconscious grammar of English, people are usually unaware of the rules for how they make sense of their relationships. For example, a couple is not aware that they have the rule, say, that if one person becomes overly clingy then the other person backs off, maintaining their comfortable level of closeness. And if that person backs off then the other person moves closer to maintain their comfortable level of closeness. The couple in this situation is non-consciously negotiating the correct level of closeness for their relationship to remain stable. Seeing the individual problem as related to the couple system is shown to increase the effectiveness of counselling, but, according to the writings of Gurman and Burton, seeing the individual in isolation requires that therapists attend to side-taking and inaccurate assessments of the systemic issues mostly because each individual is unaware of the pattern and the systemic effects of their behaviour.

In the example of the couple and of the two siblings, their actions are based on rules they are unaware of and generally believe that reality is one-sided. We all tend to feel that we see reality as it is. This is why we hear about frustration or clinginess because the individual emotion and behaviour is a signal, a communication about broken rules in the relationship. According to Watzlawick and colleagues, the attempted solution often becomes the problem because each person is inviting the other to live by a different set of rules. The solution to back off only invites more clinginess, for example, because the rule about "having distance" or "being independent" is anxiety-provoking for one of the partners. This fact refers us back to Bateson and others who discussed systemic homeostasis. The homeostasis or balance is maintained by the interpretations that people hold in the relationship and change comes with unpacking the implicit rules. With co-ordination of meaning. The reason people interpret interactions in idiosyncratic yet routine ways is linked with their history of relationships, in the family and communities in which they learnedlearnt to be themselves. Growing up in a family or society that values independence, or a family or society that discourages bonds and strong attachments, will tend to instil rules in people about not getting too close.

The Daisy Model

Communication counselling works on three levels. One is the level of how a signal or message is conveyed, another is what the signal or message is, and the other is on the level of meaning and interpretation. The daisy model is a CMM tool that brings attention to the interpretation of conversations that clients are having when they communicate with others, unravelling aspects of the reasons for interpreting and punctuating events in the way they do. In this activity, the client draws a daisy or number of daisies in which the middle represents some statement or situation, and the converging petals represent the underlying meanings, rules, and perspectives that inform it. The example given by the couple negotiating closeness is as shown in Figure 6.5.

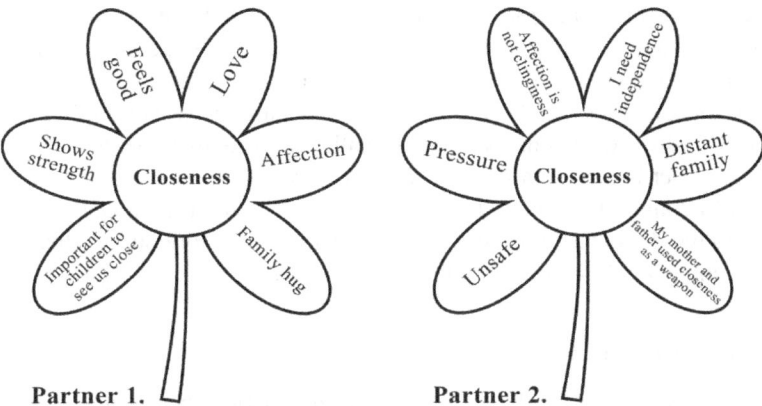

Figure 6.5 The Closeness Daisy

The word "closeness" connects to multiple words, stories, experiences, and meanings. It becomes more of a garden than a single daisy! The activity uncovers communications that are embedded into individual, couple, and family interactions. It draws attention to the episodes or differences in perspectives that generate mental health issues in clients. For one partner, closeness connects to family experiences, love, and affection. For another, it connects to rules around independence and experiences of closeness being weaponised.

Taking a second-order position is important, where we consider how the meaning of words influences how we understand clients. If I were to draw my closeness daisy, for example, the petals would have different words and different meanings attached to them. When words relate to or resemble other words or concepts in our vocabulary, Wittgenstein calls this family resemblances. That is, words connect with other words in unique ways and as counsellors we should remain aware of our ignorance of other people's resemblances. In one example of this, I led an activity for trainee counsellors called family resemblance musical chairs. We took away one chair from the circle and the standing trainee said a word, any word, such as "happy". I asked the trainee to name the first two words that came to mind when I said "happy". She said, "fun and family". I asked those who were sitting down if these were the same two words that other people had in mind, and if so, to stand up and switch seats. Out of 24 students, can you guess how many people stood up?

Zero.

We tried the activity with another word. This time, any student with one of the same connected words could stand up and switch chairs. The word was "family", and the connected words were "love and conflict". Now some people had "love" and some people had "conflict" connected to the word "family", so they moved. But nobody had the same resemblances to the word "family" or the word "happy". Thus, words do not communicate the same thing even with a shared language, culture, and subculture of trainee counsellors. From the 1900s, Wittgenstein unwittingly warned future counsellors against interfering with the resemblances of clients because we should get to know their social reality before believing we have knowledge of it. Especially in a situation like this, when clients exist in social realities that evoke painful feelings and significant mental health issues. This highlights the importance of asking questions using the specific language that clients use and asking clients to describe their reality in their own words, without suggestive language from us. In communication counselling we see meaning as personal and as such rely less on the dictionary for the meaning of words and more on the client's own embodied understanding of the vocabulary they use.

The Hierarchy of Meaning

Pearce and Cronen pushed CMM theory further than interactions between two people. They explained the ways in which society plays a defining role in how people make meaning from events, due to higher contexts. The daisy model hints towards a social context of cultural values around parenting and independence, for example. In Figure 6.6, Pearce puts forward that the content of any statement is encased in a client's "bodily sensations", which refers to how the body communicates the meaning of the words. Then there is the speech act, which Austin describes as the impact that speech has on a listener or the social world. Many people believe that speech is not a form of action, but this is incorrect. Notwithstanding threats and shouting "fire" in a crowded room, Austin examined how ordinary speech has direct consequences on the social world, and we will discuss this more in the next chapter.

The speech act is given meaning to, as discussed above, by the episode. CMM theory views the episode as contextualised within a hierarchy of meanings that includes personal and professional identity, relationship type, family experience, culture, spirituality, and politics. The meaning of a word like "closeness" or

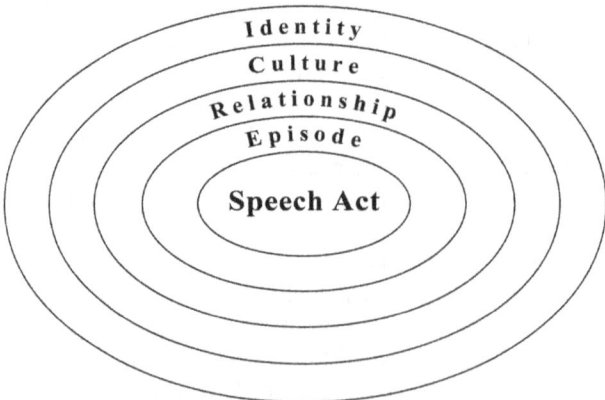

Figure 6.6 The Hierarchy of Meaning

"affection" is tied in with societal norms. These norms impose a contextual force on the meaning generated from the content of all difficulties that clients bring to therapy. People can choose their own words of course, and this demonstrates that people do have some power in the social system, but this power is limited. The implicative force is the influence that travels from individuals, couples, families, and communities up to the wider society. Movements such as gay rights and civil rights are examples of the implicative force in action, changing the social contract from the ground up, but the contextual force is stronger.

CMM states that every interaction exists within a hierarchy of meanings that contextualise how people, couples, and families experience each other, punctuate events into stories, and communicate. To reflect on the multiple meanings of client episodes, counsellors can de-construct the contexts from a communicational perspective.

The LUUUT Model

There are several communication activities available to the counsellor that unpack the higher contexts embedded in human communication and interaction. One such approach is called the LUUUT model. Let's get to know the technique by meeting a client named Martha, a 17-year-old female who came to counselling depressed, and said to me in the first session, "I am a failure".

Communication counselling involves unpacking the situation in which the statement is made, the multiple interpretations of it, and defining the episode that Martha sees herself within when making that statement in counselling. Is this statement in the episode of hope? Despair? One of loss? One of honesty?

Martha had decided not to go to university, although her family and friends had gone, and said "people who don't ... are usually failures". Martha had a full-time job in a bakery, which allowed her to continue at her ballet school. This was her life ambition. I wondered about how the episode of leaving education had influenced Martha's view of herself.

The LUUUT model helped me to focus on unheard stories. These are stories that exist for the client but that nobody appears to be listening to or paying attention to. I asked her to talk about situations where she does not feel like a failure.

Martha said her mum praised her ballet, and said she has a good chance of succeeding with her current ballet teacher. In this context, she spoke about herself as ambitious and committed, and she began to describe the context she was in as, in her words, "the bakery sacrifice". Here she felt she was sacrificing a cultural idea of success (a university education) for a personal success in dance.

Martha had found herself in the western context where "going to university is what people my age do". She felt like a failure for not sticking to this social norm. Pearce and Cronen discuss that these are the lived stories of clients' realities. Though the lived story is not the only story. There are also untold, unheard, and unknown stories. The lived, untold, unheard, unknown, and told (LUUUT) stories contextualise Martha's communication to me, and my response co-creates the ways in which she tells her story and makes meaning. Drawing attention to unheard stories can reframe how a client understands themselves.

The stories about judgement from her friends and being isolated added strength to her lived and told story. By inviting times that fight off the feeling of failure, I was challenging the unhelpful lived experience in the conversation, and she was able to tell unheard stories of success. This caused other feelings and behaviours to emerge, such as pride and commitment.

In seeing herself in the episode of "The Bakery Sacrifice", Martha constructed a more hopeful reality. A communication perspective notes that nothing innate to Martha, such as we traditionally might describe as personality, had changed. We had listened to other stories, which fed back a different self-image to her, leaving Martha feeling less like a failure and proud of herself for committing to her ballet. CMM sets out the systemic view that any change in the communication or meaning changes the problem or behaviour. In this book, we have defined the system as any stable unit maintained by on-going feedback, and here the feedback to Martha was information about unheard stories. A communication perspective sees counselling as a way of unpacking communication and providing feedback to adjust meaning.

In summary, communication theory and CMM theory sees reality as socially constructed via a layering of contexts, from politics to the culture in which it is embedded, right down to any individual emotion or perspective. How we order and punctuate events influences how we feel and behave. To change feelings and behaviours between people, a context shift or a second-order change is required, under which new possibilities in the family, peer, and social system are made. Communication counselling focuses on how people communicate, the interpersonal communication patterns, and the interpretation or meaning from which people understand one another, attempting to change the way people perceive and narrate their reality.

Further Reading

Austin, J. L. (1962). *How to do things with words*. Oxford: Clarendon.

Bateson, G. (1972). *Steps to an ecology of mind*. London: Paladin.

Bowen, M. (1985). *Family therapy in clinical practice*. Lanham, MD: Rowman and Littlefield.

Gurman, A. S., & Burton, M. (2014). Individual therapy for couple problems: Perspectives and pitfalls. *Journal of Marital and Family Therapy, 38*, 470–483. doi:10.1111/jmft.12061.

Pearce, B. (2007). *Making social worlds: A communication perspective*. Malden, MA: Blackwell Publishers.

Shannon, C., & Weaver, W. (1998). *The mathematical theory of communication*. Oxford: Marston.

Truss, L. (2007). *Eats, shoots, and leaves*. London: Harper Collins.

Watzlawick, P., Weakland, J. W., & Fisch, R. (1974). *Change*. New York: W.W. Norton & Company.

Chapter 7

Language and Discourse Counselling

The study of language began in the late 19th century, around the same time as the development of psychoanalysis. Language scientists became known as linguists, and they opened up a whole field of scientific investigation. Linguistics and psychotherapy remained out of touch for much of their early lifespan. Ludwig Wittgenstein, a mathematician considered to be one of the great founders of the linguistics movement, originally saw language as a sound-based system for referring to objects in the world. Each vibrating air molecule, travelling from deep within the vocal cords onto the thin cone-shaped membrane of the eardrum, was viewed as carrying information about something real and something tangible. This defined language as a communication system in which words referred to real objects like cats, dogs, rivers, and pineapples.

In the decades that followed, Wittgenstein came to strongly disagree with his younger self. He noticed that words in a language did not always correspond to objects in the real world. And that words were active; words did things in the social world. They charm, they bite, they hurt, they heal. When studied closely, language looked more like a social tool. Over the next hundred years, language and social scientists studied the effects of seeing language as a social utensil, and their findings were translated into language and discourse psychotherapies. This chapter examines the modern theory of language and how findings from linguistics have been converted into a counselling approach.

Spoken Language

Language is a pronounceable sound or vocal pattern that carries meaning. In communication theory, language can be used for communication when one person makes sounds and utterances in such a way that influences or affects another person. The linguist Noam Chomsky makes the controversial yet quite factual claim that there is no such thing as a national language, like English or Chinese, not really. When linguists study the details, there are only different ways of speaking that are more or less similar. When two people have high similarity in their vocal patterns, they can communicate through language. Having the shared sound for "hello" allows meaning to be transferred quickly between two people of the same

DOI: 10.4324/9781003480808-8

language community. With spoken and written language, communication becomes optimal because there is less ambiguity in words than in grunts and howls.

Take any so-called national language such as English. It's straightforward to visualise how English varies from the north to the south, from the housing estate to the royal estate, and from the dentist's chair to the psychotherapist's couch. Each way of speaking, each accent and word-bank or vocabulary, communicates something vaguely English that would seem unintelligible in Shakespearean England or medieval times. Or even in contemporary times when older people try to communicate with younger people. Language is not a fixed thing that can be trapped inside a dictionary, although many people try. Language is an everchanging convention of spoken, written, and signed symbols used by social groups to communicate and organise themselves. But even this definition is unhelpful! Language is mostly sub-vocal, said inside your own head. As such, language plays a deep role in your private psychological life. I'm guessing, for example, that you're reading this inside your head rather than reading it out loud!

The Science of Language

The kind of vocabulary and accent that each person uses is broken down by linguistics into a variety of categories. The sounds come under "phonetics". The words come under "lexicon" or vocabulary. The sentences come under "grammar". The meaning of the words and sentences when put together with grammar is "semantics". And the use of the language in a social context is "pragmatics". These are the categories most important for this chapter, but many linguistic features exist outside of these categories.

For a counsellor, these language categories separate different levels of meaning from the client's words and utterances. For example, there is an interesting phenomenon at the minute that is challenging the counselling community. Therapy gurus and self-help hacks are distorting findings from psychology to sell alternative therapies to unsuspecting people. In the year of writing, the term "counsellor", the term "psychotherapist", and the term "psychologist" are not protected titles like "children and young people's counsellor", "systemic psychotherapist", and "counselling psychologist". Many unqualified people make money from unknowing clients without the correct training and supervision under some version of the name "therapist" or "counsellor". Often when I see and hear alternative counsellors, I notice how well they do on the phonetic level. That is, the sounds they produce are often inviting, engaging, and therapeutic. Yet, on the semantic level, what they are saying is often meaningless or misconstrued.

A trained counsellor being phonetically good but semantically bad is okay when clients feel the words as useful rather than understanding them intellectually. Empathic words that aren't fully coherent semantically can be of use in the same way that counsellors probe into semantically sound words like "I'm okay" when the sounds or phonetics of those words are incongruent emotionally. This multi-level communication is possible because of how our brains decode the different

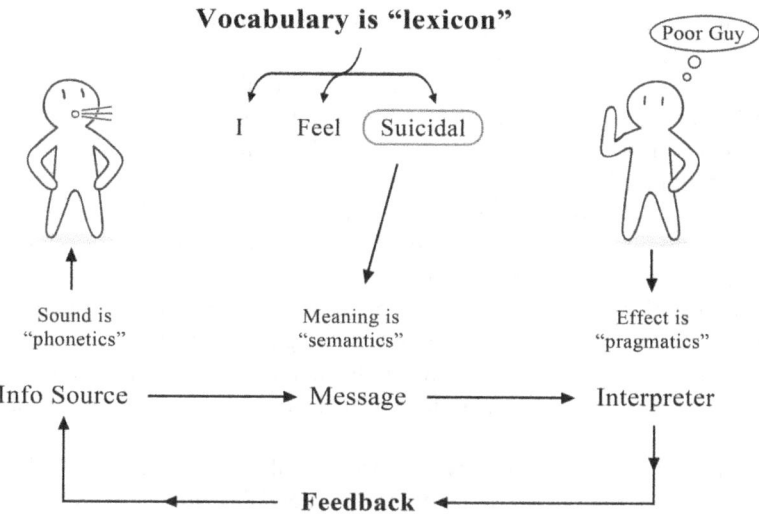

Figure 7.1 The Linguistics of Client Statements

sound, word, grammatical, and semantic elements of language. Norbert Wiener, the cybernetics theorist, noticed that decoding language happens mostly in the listener's head rather than in the information carried by the words or sounds. This means that the listener receives less information than the speaker sends, and the listener models the speaker's mind or meaning within her own brain. Her memory and prior experience fill the gaps of information and translate the sound into complex ideas, intentions, and meanings.

Let's look at a clinical example.

For the first time in two months of counselling, a 31-year-old male mentioned the word "suicide". He said he's had suicidal thoughts for around one year and, as he spoke this, he laughed, uncomfortably. The linguistically aware counsellor focuses on the sound and contradiction of the laugh, the sound and meaning of the statement, and the pragmatics (the social effect) of having mentioned suicide two months into counselling and not at the beginning (see Figure 7.1). Intuitively we know that the person feels awkward or embarrassed about having held their life so fragile in the palm of their hand.

The Daisy-Chain Model

In the previous chapter, we introduced the daisy model: a way of unpacking the meaning behind a word. From a semantic or meaning perspective, the daisy model takes important words and unravels their meaning. This allows clients to make meaning out of their experiences. The daisy model supports clients to consider, on the language level, how they co-ordinate their meanings with others pragmatically. Many unhealthy interpersonal patterns can be explained by unpacking the meaning of the words that each person exchanges in their separate vocabularies. The same words don't always have the same meaning.

In the daisy-chain activity, the client was asked to draw a daisy with the word "suicide" in the inside disc of the flower. Then the client connected words that described thoughts, experiences, problems, and other aspects of their suicidality (Figure 7.2).

Now the counsellor pushes the activity further to support the client in creating a daisy chain. This consists of one of two things. The first might be taking the word from any petal and creating a new but connected daisy (Figure 7.3). Conversations about connected words reveal a semantic chain, a connected series of meanings that enrich the description of the problem. In many cases it reveals hopeful words. Peter Lang, one of the early pioneers of systemic trainings in the United Kingdom, said that every problem is a frustrated dream. In this daisy chain, the client is connecting with a desire for relief. Most people who feel suicidal actually don't want to die, they want relief.

The final part of the daisy-chain activity is to draw the imagined daisies, the internalised daisies, for significant people in the client's relationship systems (Figure 7.4). This invites the client to think about a friend, a parent, a colleague, and so on, in terms of what imagined petals they would write in connecting to the word "suicide". Here the client reflects on the meaning of their presenting problem or their psychological vocabulary to others, connecting with their truths and their realities. If the client discovers what they mean to other people in their life, this could be the difference between making a life-or-death decision. The underpinning systemic theory is that the client is, in the words of the inventor of the reflecting team, Tom Andersen, reflecting on their systems of meaning. Many clients widen their perspective on the problem by using the daisy-chain model to work on the semantics of the words they use. The process of drawing tends to be relaxing for the client and slows down the meaning-making process to deepen the reflective process.

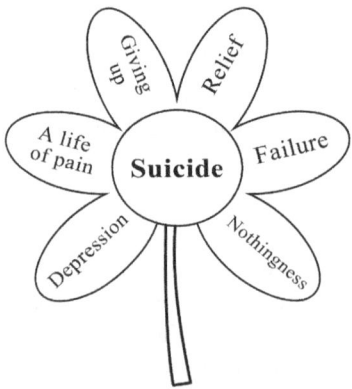

Figure 7.2 Daisy-Chain Example

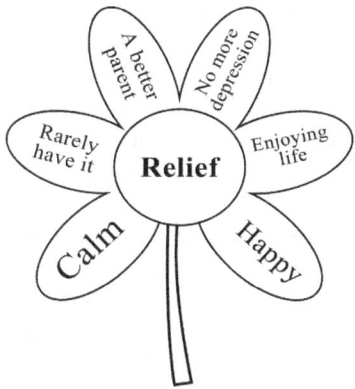

Figure 7.3 "Relief" Daisy Chain

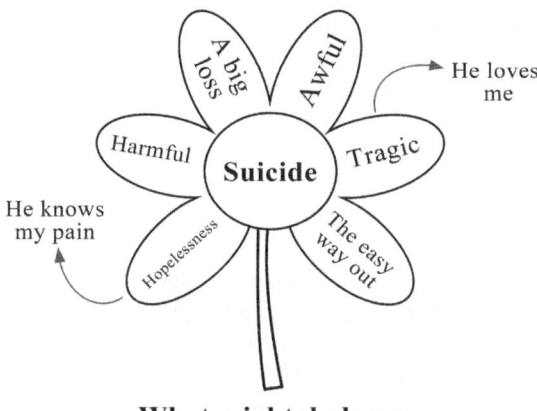

What might dad say.

Figure 7.4 "Father's" Daisy Chain

Speech Act Theory

Important support for language and meaning-making as a legitimate form of counselling came from sociologists and linguists who attempted, and struggled, to define the difference between speech and an action. That speech creates social realities means that words are far from harmless. They scar, provoke, enchant, and soothe, and can have dramatically inspiring and life-saving effects on people. Let's consider a typical situation in which a word constitutes an action. In a court of law, the judge exclaims "Guilty!". In this situation, police officers around the identified "defendant", equipped with handcuffs and heavy police batons, respond by escorting the newly identified "prisoner" to a nearby cell.

In this example, language is flexible. It both communicates information and directly changes the physical world. Namely, that the word "guilty" changed a free man into a prisoner. In this scenario, the word counted as an action. JL Austin developed this observation into his iconic Speech Act Theory, in which speech is shown to perform actions when there is an accepted conventional procedure. If I shout "guilty" at the person who cut me up in traffic this morning, sadly, the full force of the law does not apply.

Speech acts are most visible in legally sanctioned institutions such as in marriage and sports, for example, but are part of every social context. People's behaviour sits within a typical range of acceptable conventions, traditions, and social norms. Behaviours that stray from acceptable ranges are in some way discouraged through feedback (usually verbal language or body language) such as scorn, humiliation, anger, legislation and even medication or counselling. The most common example in psychiatry is the use of diagnosis that takes a client or patient and defines them as disordered or as mentally unwell. Diagnosis comes with legal sanctions, rights, and sometimes intrusive social practices. The counselling modality is also a social convention that uses words to act on the social world. In one modality, a person's anxiety is due to low self-awareness and acceptance, yet, in another modality, the same facts are labelled as unconscious desires or defence mechanisms. If you watch a counsellor with either of these approaches in mind, you will see them act differently in response to the client.

Linguistic Relativity

For many people, a strawman argument comes into view here. This is an argument that takes something like social constructionism and attributes claims to it that were never made, burning the metaphorical strawman, the false claim, instead of the real claim of the theory. Many people feel that there are "facts" like being person-centred, using diagnosis, having depression, and being psychotic. They will say that the words have not created something but that something, an anxiety disorder, or an autism spectrum disorder, existed and was innocently labelled by the terminology of the psychiatrist and the counsellor.

It is a respectable view that diagnoses and counselling formulations exist as a matter of labelling. The social constructionist does not deny the reality of someone feeling panicked about going outside and sweating at the thought of social interaction. The theory draws attention to how the act of naming is itself a construction, a way of perceiving those things as a pattern, often in a way that helps and often in a way that stigmatises people. Cognitive scientists such as Lera Boroditsky have shown that the way we label our world changes the way we perceive it. This theory of linguistic relativity, in which the way we speak about our world alters our perception, is the basis of a systemic social constructionist model of counselling. That is, how we and clients speak about the world influences their mental distress. Calling the above situation "general anxiety disorder" could have the social effect of bringing the person some support. It could also have the effect of having them interpret themselves as dysfunctional and incapable. A systemic approach tries to find the right language to empower clients.

Systems Theory and Dominant Discourses

How does systems theory, which views counselling problems as formed from patterns of interactions, fit with the idea that language impacts mental health? Well, since a system is a set of things working together as part of a network, the actions of any individual member can be viewed as part of a sequence of interactions, supporting the steady state of the system, which we have called its homeostasis. In 1948, when Wiener coined the term "cybernetics" to define the science of systems, he described a stable system as any system that maintains its homeostasis using feedback loops in a way that is self-stabilising. The concept of stabilisation through verbal feedback loops is important here. The philosopher Michel Foucault examined the structure of social systems and discovered that language is a powerful and continuous set of feedback loops that societies use to remain intact. His famous idea that knowledge is power is often misunderstood. He did not mean that knowing more equates to being more powerful. He meant that the capacity to create knowledge indicates a person's power.

Knowledge is created through social discourse. In a rousing book called *Madness and Civilisation*, Foucault explored how words and ways of speaking about mental health are tied up with political power. At one end of the spectrum was the definition of a healthy person. The definition of mental illness served the function of validating some ways of behaving as normal and others abnormal, and people have a tendency to fit in with social norms. Thus, creating knowledge about what constitutes the most acceptable and unacceptable type of person plays into how people from different communities experience themselves. Social discourse creates knowledge and power over people.

Most of us are unconscious of just how our identity is tied up with what Foucault called the dominant discourse, which is a vocabulary about a specific aspect of society that most people use to create and uphold the social norms. For instance, the dominant discourse that men should not show weakness and women should not show anger exists subtly in terminology like "man-bag" and "guy-liner". This is because on the one hand these terms imply the social norm for handbags and eye make-up is that women should use these products. The concept of femininity as being linked with beauty implies an ideology that upholds males in positions of strength and power. It takes millions of people hundreds of years to change the dominant discourse, and usually through countless horrific deaths and abuses of power. In itself, the word "man-bag" is of course one tiny part of a bigger social dialogue. When adding up all the words the counselling client uses to express their reality, it becomes possible to deconstruct their social identity into distinct categories and discourses.

The Social GGRRAACCEESS

A systemic way of unpacking dominant discourses in counselling is using a model designed by husband-and-wife team Alison Roper-Hall and John Burnham. They developed a mnemonic for helping counsellors and clients to examine different social discourses that intrude on client perceptions. They noticed that in counselling, the most common dominant discourses are linked with a person's gender identity, geography, race, religion, age, ability, class, culture, education, ethnicity, sexual identity, and spirituality. Hence, the terminology for this was the social GGRRAACCEESS. Since then, an extra "s" has been added, which stands for "something else" important to the client. By exploring social graces, the counsellor helps the client develop meaning and ways of gaining power over the discourses that guide their actions.

Bird's-Eye View

The systemic supervisor and author Johnella Bird developed a useful reflective activity relevant to the social graces. She used it to help her supervisees construct narratives. We can transfer her approach to counselling, taking a Bird's-eye view, by helping clients construct and reflect on narratives about their social graces. She encourages counsellors to:

a)   Identify the beliefs that clients hold
b)   Express these beliefs in reflective language
c)   Locate and explore these beliefs in context
d)   Reflect on the effects of these beliefs in particular circumstances

A case example can highlight the importance of this approach. The client is a male in his early 30s having recently separated from his long-term girlfriend. In taking a Bird's-eye view, we look out for the problem or the hope the client is bringing. He tells us that he has been feeling low in mood and isolated. We show systemic curiosity towards the client's difficulties, exploring discourses that connect with his social graces. He tells us that being a single man in his early 30s is like a "social death sentence". A counsellor interested in dominant discourses would highlight at least three important social graces. "He" tells us something about gender. "Single man" refers us to dominant discourses around sexuality and social norms. "Early 30s" brings in conversations around the social expectations of age. Taking each GRACE separately, we support the client to:

a)   Identify the beliefs he holds about being 30
b)   Express these beliefs in reflective language
c)   Locate and explore these beliefs in context
d)   Reflect on the effects of these beliefs in particular circumstances

Social discourses around the client's age assume he should be in a stable relationship, own his own home, and be advanced in his career. None of these things are true of this client. The dominant discourse therefore creates power over him because it is used to evaluate his worthiness. Despite having a good friendship group, isolation seems the only option when he doesn't fit in with the social norms. Although he is physically present, he feels socially excluded. When these beliefs play out in his social circle, his friends unknowingly create feelings of failure in him. Feedback loops come in the form of questions, comments, and actions. For instance, they ask him if he's met any love interests. When answering "no", he is jokingly patronised by being given dating advice. Also, the client sees many of his friends having children, getting married, and getting a mortgage. The parties and social gatherings that hang around these social milestones contribute further to his negative self-evaluation. And the effects of these beliefs and discourses are that the client creates a negative self-image, and he sinks into a low mood.

At this point, we invite the client to reflect on other social graces. This time the client highlights his gender as important. We:

a)   Identify the beliefs he holds about being male
b)   Express these beliefs in reflective language
c)   Locate and explore these beliefs in context
d)   Reflect on the effects of these beliefs in particular circumstances

The client's gender comes with constraining dominant discourses. Men are not socially permitted to display sadness. He feels he must put on a brave and supportive face socially, affirming the things that create a sense of failure for him. These beliefs are affirmed when he does show moments of sadness. For example, when he mentioned feeling rubbish to a friend, he was playfully teased. The client is clear that his friends are supportive. He trusts them. But being male and showing emotions is met with social feedback that undermines or pushes aside the emotion. Systemically, we could have punctuated this differently and said that his socially uncomfortable emotion evokes his friends' dismissive responses. One effect of this is that he shows shyness and a lack of self-belief in reaching out for emotional support. Coming to counselling felt like the only option.

Intersectionality

The multiple layers of identity are summed up in a concept called intersectionality. Human identity is layered or intersectional in that age, sexuality, and gender are intersecting parts of a person's identity. In the intersectional way of thinking, the lower emotional expressiveness of men is primarily about stacking up multiple social discourses, adding social graces together into a unique self-identity. When a social system constructs value judgements about different identities, people develop mental health problems when their intersecting social graces are disadvantaged by that system. In this way, emotional health reflects social justice. Counselling is political.

With the male client experiencing low mood, Foucault would say that the power over him is that the social system has produced knowledge and meaning to exclude his form of existence. This is a rather potent statement. Counsellors use the strength of this concept, of discourse power, to continue to tap into the identities that empower clients. Or they help him to challenge the social discourse. In some cases, counselling serves as a form of support for someone to conform to social norms. This depends on how useful conformity is for the client.

With our client in mind, let's imagine that we invite a third set of reflections using Johnella Bird's four questions. We ask him to reflect on "something else" that gives him a positive sense of himself. He says the identity in which he feels most competent is "being a manager". In hearing this positive social grace, we:

a)   Identified the beliefs he held about being a manager
b)   Asked him to express the beliefs in reflective language
c)   Located and explored his beliefs about being a manager in context
d)   Reflected on the effects of his beliefs in particular circumstances

As a manager, the client is emotionally expressive, nurturing, and empathic. For instance, a supervisee was on leave from work following a family bereavement. The client showed compassion and gave him additional time off for the grieving process. He wrote to the employee personally, and the employee was very appreciative in his response. Using Bird's model, alongside the social graces, enabled the client to reflect on restrictive dominant discourses and challenge them by considering intersectionality. When reflecting on his identity as a manager, he felt he had more in common with his successful friends and was able to consider ways to bring his managerial set of skills into his personal life. He decided to resist, uncomfortably at first, the belief that he cannot tell his friends about emotional difficulties. And unsurprisingly his friends welcomed his hidden feelings with compassion. From my reading of his heightened confidence in seeing his friends and being more open about his feelings, I took away a change in his discourse about friendship. If a friend cares about you, they will rewrite the social contract in favour of your emotional health.

Second-Order Change in Discourse

Language and discourse counselling makes the prediction that people change their mindset when they unpack restrictive beliefs and values. In a sense this brings about an idea that is quite profound. In every moment, a person can decide who they are. Although we are all constrained by social discourse, our creativity is also an ally in rewriting our self-identity. If, systemically, two people's interactions uphold dominant discourses, then two or more people's interactions can reconstruct dominant discourses within the boundaries of their relationship (Table 7.1).

As we have seen in previous chapters, systems theory states that for a system—such as a friendship system—to undergo changes in the patterns of interaction,

Table 7.1 Dominant Discourses in Social Interaction

Client	Interaction	Friend
Dominant discourse: Men do not show feelings **Action:** Reservedly shows sadness		**Dominant discourse:** Men do not show feelings **Action:** Minimises feelings by saying, sarcastically, "cheer up!"
Alternative discourse: Friends are compassionate **Action:** Explains that they are struggling to show sadness		**Alternative discourse:** Friends are compassionate **Action:** Encourages feelings compassionately

a second-order change must occur. This is a change in the rules governing the friendship system. The difference in rules relates to how the friendship is socially constructed from information that emerges out of dominant discourses in the wider society. Societal beliefs about companions, boys, feelings, and so on, contextualise interaction patterns and dictate a framework for individual turn-taking, like shying away from feelings or harmlessly ridiculing a friend's sadness.

Individual psychology becomes a concept that strips the individual of the multiple contexts in which they exist. In systems theory, individual behaviours make sense as part of relationships. Therefore, the emotionally withdrawn male operates inside a wider social system where gender, geography, race, religion, age, ability, class, culture, education, ethnicity, sexuality, and spirituality become the database from which cultural information shapes the discourse that motivates his behaviour.

In theory, any person can instigate a change in the rules of the friendship game, by behaving differently. This first-order change will often be responded to in a first-order way. That is, with behaviour that limits the change to fit with the underlying social rules. Complementary escalation, where the more one person does one behaviour, the more another does a different behaviour, is explained very well by discourse theory. If we see the friendship as being glued together by the rule "we keep things light and don't discuss serious feelings" then the more one person attempts to do so, the more the other will prevent it. Often until the relationship breaks down. In this case, ridicule serves the function of keeping the friendship stable. It complements the behaviour that challenges the underlying rules. But stability means upholding a dominant discourse that challenges the happiness of the friendship. In cases such as this, the client talking about the talk, or talking about the rules of the friendship, can create a change in the definition of their relationship: this is a second-order change.

Social movements are premised on the friction that is created in relationships of social injustice. Racism, sexism, ableism are all examples where citizens with enough time-elapsed and social discrimination create a swell of interactions that begin to challenge the status quo. Slowly over time the society changes its dominant discourses. What is acceptable today may look abhorrent to a future society.

Positioning Theory

This is the final section of the chapter. Here we think about the way that language and social context establish positions for clients and people when they communicate. Interpersonal communication and language put people into contexts that are difficult to shake off. When the client is positioned into a lifestyle or backed into an emotional corner that restricts them, inevitably, problems surface.

Here I am talking about positioning theory. And let's consider a counselling situation to illustrate the idea.

Recently I phoned an adoptive mother-of-two to discuss a referral from the GP. The client, Sam, is an eight-year-old boy who lives with his biological sister (Jess, five) and adoptive parents (Lynn and Gary) in a small English town. He was referred for individual therapy following an assault that occurred by Sam against his younger sister. The referrer was the family GP and he requested individual support to reduce Sam's anger and violence, and to increase his "emotional management" (Figure 7.5).

When accepting individual referrals for clients such as Sam, positioning theory is a useful way to consider how the referrer's request positions me towards Sam, Sam towards me, me towards the family, and the family towards Sam. Positioning theory was developed in social psychology. Rom Harré and Luk Van Langenhove describe a position as the rights and allowances that someone is afforded within a social context. The positions available to men and women, for example, are different. The social space gives and takes away rights and expectations. Speech acts, which we discussed earlier in the chapter, position people into a storyline that fits

Lynn   Gary

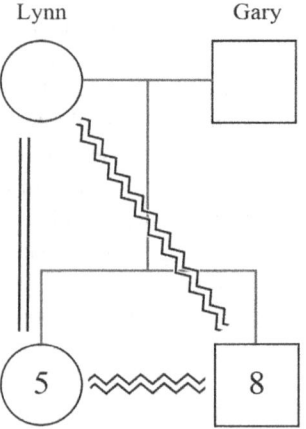

Figure 7.5 Sam's Genogram

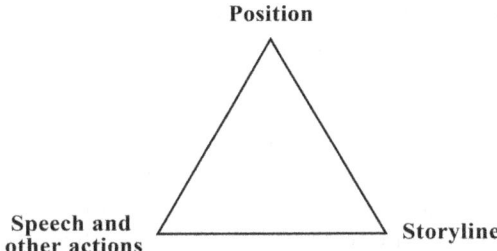

Figure 7.6 The Positioning Triangle

the social norms. By talking to someone, or even by ignoring them, you are inviting them into a social position. How does Sam's referral form position me? What language did it use to create a storyline for me to accept?

The Positioning Triangle

The referral language located the problem within Sam (his anger) and suggested the solution as linked with his actions (his emotional management). Often positioning creates a tension between therapists and referred children because the actions of the family are usually part of how the child makes sense of their behaviour. Systemically, childhood anger is a problem within the relationships between children, family, and social systems rather than individuals alone. According to Harré and Langenhove, social positions are always disputable. And this has positive effects for our clients when we unpack social discourse and interpersonal patterns. The storyline evoked by the referral can be accepted or adapted by the counsellor in how they speak and act towards the client (Figure 7.6).

In Sam's case, positioning theory encouraged me to shift from an individual approach to a family approach. This was the first action towards addressing the individualistic gender discourse that was positioning me towards seeing the problem within the child. Accepting the terms of any referral can be harmful to the process of change when it reinforces the social patterns that brought about the problem.

Harré and Langenhove define positioning as "the discursive construction of personal stories that make a person's actions intelligible" (p. 16). By discursive construction they mean that in social interaction people take up and invite others into roles within personal and cultural stories. Dominant discourses play out through social interaction and limit the available positions. During dialogue, people position themselves and others within certain meaning-laden stories that maintain their group identities.

Gender Positioning

The language of the parent and the counsellor can invite a "boy" or a "girl" into gender positions. The children's language can take up, reject, or re-construct certain positions, and each utterance in the talk is an act of positioning and repo-sitioning, which maintains the dominant discourse around gender. It is clear that English society socialises people into a binary view of gender. When a child acts in the social world, he or she is taught to understand his or her actions according to being a "he" or a "she". Males are positioned as having to prove their masculinity. Boys are encouraged to be macho and to physicalise instead of to verbalise their needs. The anthropologist Kate Fox studied English male emotions and found that "English males are allowed to express only three emotions" (p. 243), which are the emotions of surprise, elation/triumph, and anger.

Negative responses follow non-masculine expressions of emotion. This can be seen as positioning males as having the right to a limited range of emotional expressions. Therefore, considering how clients are positioned within gender dis-course can contribute to a reduction of gendered behaviours such as anger.

Acknowledging the Current Positions

I booked to see Sam at home. When I arrived at the house, Sam's younger sister Jess answered the door with their mother. Sam waited angrily with his back to me in the living room. The father Gary was unable to attend due to work commitments. Take a moment to consider, what positions were available, what positions were taken up, and what storylines were we creating?

Through the lens of positioning theory, we see how the two females took on the social lead for convening the counselling system, and the two males were absenting themselves. Such a positioning of masculine and feminine roles can be understood even ahead of the interactions. For instance, to schedule the counselling session I had called the mother, not the father, and so I had positioned the parents into gender roles already. My bias towards calling the mother, whose number was the only one on the referral form, was influenced by the GP and the wider cultural assumptions about mothers being the main carers of children.

Entering the living room, Sam's physical behaviour was verbalised by the two females (his mother and sister). They interpreted his physical display as him not wanting to be there, him being "moody", and him disliking talking. The process of the females talking about emotional communication and positioning the boy as the object of the emotional communication reinforced the cultural ideologies around gender. Sam began to bang his fists on the armchair in front of him, and he remained with his back turned to us.

Intentional Positioning

Most positioning is tacit positioning: learnt and automatic everyday interactions that come to be experienced as normal. Intentional positioning is when the coun-sellor actively challenges a tacit position perceived to be unhelpful. Counsellors can use words and actions to create different positions within the discourse. For instance, in responding to the mother and sister, I questioningly replied, "moody?

… I guess having someone come to bother you at home could do that … You said, talking? … I brought some things to play with if none of you feel like talking".

My intention was to respect the words of the mother-daughter family subgroup but to vary them in the direction, not of Sam's behaviour problems, but of my role in having positioned Sam into a difficult conversation. This allowed Sam out of the trap of being positioned as the problem.

As a second act of intentional positioning, I walked away from Sam towards a photo of Gary on the wall. I asked Lynn and Jess if this was "dad", while Sam inspected the game I had left on the floor. The intention was to re-frame our inter-action as centred on the family and not Sam, while communicating that the session can be flexible to his needs. The position I hoped to invite was that we were all con-nected through our behaviours rather than being organised by Sam. It is important to highlight that males hold most of the power in British society, but in verbal com-munication processes male children are often disadvantaged and can communicate such disadvantage with what looks to be moodiness, reluctance, and controlling behaviour. By re-positioning the whole session into a family activity, we generated a big change in Sam's engagement. Sam's engagement and his disengagement can be better understood relationally by considering how gender discourse was unin-tentionally positioning us. As the session started, Sam's anger disappeared.

The Positioning Compass

The positioning compass can help clients learn about the positions they take up when interacting with others. There are hundreds of thousands of words in the English language and each word has the potential to be important. Karen Partridge, the systemic psychotherapist and clinical psychologist who developed the tool, explains that important or rich words are crucial to take hold of in counselling. The therapist supports the client to draw a straight line between rich words and their opposite. This creates a spectrum-line between two different positions. Taking more resonant words and their opposites allows the client to draw a compass of positions, something that looks a bit like a dandelion head, with each spectrum-line passing through a centre point.

The meaning of each of the client's words reveals something about their social identity. Probing into the meaning of each word sets the client on an adventure for researching their perspective and experience. Taking a rich word from Sam's fam-ily, "anger", we can ask the person who spoke this word about its meaning and its opposite meaning. We might draw the line shown in Figure 7.7.

The positioning compass reflects on the client's problem by deconstructing desirable and undesirable social positions. To someone in the family, the opposite of anger is being calm. In unpacking these words, a counsellor explores when anger

Calmness 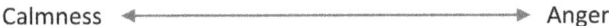 Anger

Figure 7.7 Calmness–Anger Polar Positioning

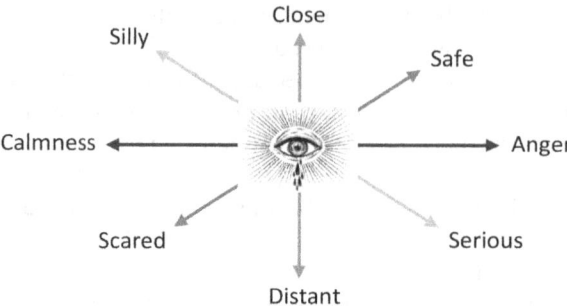

Figure 7.8 Sam's Family Compass

and when calmness happens. They can ask, where on the spectrum are you today? Why is calmness important to you? With an individual or a family, different words can be mined for their hidden hopes and dreams. A reminder of what Peter Lang used to say, "Every problem is a frustrated dream".

The metaphor of the compass is poignant. Karen Partridge sees this approach as helping a client to find themselves. By stepping into the clients' words, lingering on the meaning of their statements, we allow their ideas, experiences, and feelings to orient us as the counsellor in the therapeutic conversation. Stories begin to emerge. Often the reason for the richness of a word is a background story of pain or rejection. Sometimes the opposite of a rich word is a motivating force, other times it's a stick that has been used to coerce clients into taking up certain positions. Karen likes to draw an eye in the middle of the compass, to encourage clients to see from the middle of two positions, impartially. This gives clients a greater vantage point on themselves, their families, and their social environment (see Figure 7.8).

Having family members position themselves on the compass was useful in unpacking how they positioned one another. The work with Sam and his family began to unpack the social discourse and positions that characterised their family system. One of the ideas that sprang from work around the positioning power of dominant discourses was narrative therapy, and the work with Sam and his family followed in this direction. For that reason, we are going to end the chapter here and pick up the rest of the family story in the next section that introduces narrative and story counselling.

Further Reading

Anderson, T. (1995). *Reflecting processes; Acts of informing and forming. You can borrow my eyes but you must not take them away from me!* New York: The Guilford Press.

Austin, J. L. (1962). *How to do things with words.* Oxford: Clarendon.

Boroditsky, L., Schmidt, L., & Phillips, W. (2003). Sex, syntax, and semantics. In D. Gentner & S. Goldin-Meadow (Eds.), *Language in mind: Advances in the study of language and cognition* (pp. 61–79). Cambridge, MA: MIT Press.

Burnham, J. (2012). Developments in social GRRRAAACCEEESSS: Visible—invisible and voiced—Unvoiced. In I.-B. Krause (Ed.), *Mutual perspectives: Culture and reflexivity in contemporary systemic psychotherapy* (pp. 139–160). London: Karnac.

Chomsky, N. (2006). *Language and mind* (3rd ed.). Cambridge: Cambridge University Press. doi:10.1017/CBO9780511791222.

Foucault, M. (1965). *Madness and civilisation: A history of insanity in the age of reason.* New York: Pantheon Books.

Fox, K. (2004). *Watching the English, the hidden rules of English behaviour.* London: Hodder and Stoughton.

Harré, R., & Van Langenhove, L. (Eds.). (1999). *Positioning theory.* Oxford: Blackwell.

Hornsby, D. (2014). *Linguistics, a complete introduction.* London: Hodder and Stoughton.

Lang, P., & McAdam, E. (1997). Narrative-ating: Future dreams in present living, jottings on an honouring theme. *Human Systems: The Journal of Systemic Consultation and Management, 8*(1), 3–12.

Lang, P., & McAdam, E. (2009). *Appreciative work in schools.* West Sussex: Kingsham Press.

Partridge, K. (2007). The positioning compass: A tool to facilitate reflexive positioning. *Human Systems: The Journal of Systemic Consultation and Management, 18,* 96–111.

Wittgenstein, L. (1953). *Philosophical investigations.* Oxford: Blackwell.

Chapter 8

Narrative and Story Counselling

In the previous chapter we saw how language supplies social power to speakers and listeners. We found out that speech is equivalent to action when social norms permit it to be. Speech and vocabulary conspire together to create dominant discourses about social identity. The dramatic effects of social discourse cannot be understated for their psychological effects on people. Human systems generate culture and social values in which conversation drives people into social positions, and this chapter presents the narrative theories and techniques that have emerged to attend to the impact of stories on counselling clients.

Michael White and David Epston, two practical systemic theorists, noticed that systemic theories did not account for all features of how clients socially constructed meaning from relationships. They observed that people who come to therapy are often objectified by discourse and carry pathologising discourse around with them inside their self-image. That is, when a conversation becomes weighted towards a person's psychological baggage, the person begins to live inside a disparaging identity. People's lives become storied by societal ideals and, according to White and Epston, counselling is a place for unravelling totalising stories. That is, counselling unravels stories that have been acting like total descriptions of clients.

The culmination of systems theory, social constructionism, linguistics, positioning theory, and the theory of dominant discourses led White and Epston to the idea of narrative therapy. They define a narrative as a spoken or written account that connects events into a story. Interpersonal patterns create stories that set the context for how people relate to one another.

Sam's Family Session

Returning to the family from the previous chapter, in which Sam was the identified client, we can understand the theory behind narrative therapy in more detail. After we had re-positioned the counselling as a family activity, we played a family game, which was to build a marble rollercoaster. This positioned Sam as the leader. He became vocal, and even more so than his mother and sister. Sam began to build part of the rollercoaster. His sister struggled to attach the parts and tipped her section over in frustration. This interaction led Jess to cross her arms and refuse to go on.

DOI: 10.4324/9781003480808-9

Sam showed Jess how to attach the track. His sister and mother did not respond to him, and Sam leant in and raised his voice. As before, his sister and mother tried to resolve the issue without responding to Sam, and Sam threw a piece of the track at his sister. Jess began to cry, and Lynn suggested that Sam had a time-out.

Sam's frustration was responded to like a plot point in their family script; it was sanctioned. On the other hand, Jess's frustration was responded to with support and understanding. Sam's behaviour positioned his mother and sister as much or as little as their behaviour positioned him, but in all this positioning certain narratives were heard and others were muted. Narrative therapy considers the stories that are being created through the family's interaction, or any social interaction, and it highlights muted stories that generate change.

> [Me]: Sam, I think your sister gets scared when you shout at her, and your mum gets scared when you throw things. Before that, you tried to say something, could you try and say it again but calmer so your mum and sister can hear you?

Sam explained that he wanted to show his sister how to fit the track together. I wondered out loud how he could show his sister how the track works without becoming angry. His mother Lynn looked unsure about allowing this to happen, since he had just been aggressive. Nonetheless Lynn encouraged Jess to go and sit with Sam to learn about making the track. Jess sat on Sam's lap, and he hugged her while he explained how to fit the track together. Jess, being five, continued to hold the pieces upside down, and Sam laughed and tickled her while showing her how to fit the pieces together properly. They were able to build the track together, and they made quick progress in building two layers of their rollercoaster.

This first intervention appeared to generate a shift in the siblings' relationship. From Lynn's point of view, it looked markedly different. I had observed a change in Sam, but his mother had not observed a change. This prompted Lynn to encourage Sam to stop hugging Jess.

A Second-Order Perspective

Lynn's response confused me. It highlighted that I needed to consider what Von Foerster referred to as second-order cybernetics. That is, it was crucial for me to consider my role in having constructed the events into a storyline or narrative about change. In my storyline, Lynn's response signalled her as being the problem because she disqualified the therapeutic change in Sam. This idea ran very closely to my family script! I have a historic bias towards seeing mothers as responsible for children's emotional problems, connected to my personal experiences of being a child in my family and to the wider social discourse around being male. Personal narratives can colour therapeutic encounters and it's important we take a second-order position.

I encouraged Lynn to reflect out loud on what she was observing. This was in order to understand how she narrated the events. Lynn said that while the hugging looked nice, it was Sam's way of gaining control over his sister, and this could turn into violence. I asked Lynn to teach me how to spot the difference between affection that is risky and affection that is safe. The word "teach" was intended as positioning the parent as the knowledge-holder, thus reducing my power as the male therapist, which may have been a barrier to co-ordinating our two points of view. I learned that while I was in the frame of harmonious-sibling-relationships (and I get along with my siblings!), Lynn was in the frame of protecting a vulnerable girl from a violent boy. In the narrative frame of protection, sibling affection looks suspicious and risky. Lynn said that if Sam lets Jess go when she wants to get off his lap, then this would be a sign that he is being affectionate rather than controlling. Our co-construction of the storyline now allowed for a "controlling" narrative frame and an "affection" narrative frame according to how the children continued with their interaction.

[Me]: "Jess, would you and Sam pause a moment? I would like to ask what you thought about what your brother did just now." When Sam and Jess paused, I asked Jess about her brother's actions. I asked her what she would call the action her brother took in the previous moment. She said "kind". I asked what affect him being kind had on her. She said she had more "fun". I asked Jess if she noticed anything different about Sam when he was having "fun" and being "kind"; she said he was more "silly", and she laughed.

I turned to Sam and asked what he hoped his mother would think or feel when she saw him being kind or fun. He said he did not know (probably a complicated question for an eight-year-old!). I tried again and asked him what it was like when his mum saw him being kind. He said he "felt better". This encouraged Lynn, Sam, and Jess into the "affection/kind" narrative of Sam and Jess's relationship. Lynn responded to her children's words by passing rollercoaster pieces over to Sam, while Jess remained on Sam's lap. Lynn's actions symbolised that change had been generated in the narrative frame she used to interpret Sam's behaviour. And the game continued and ended without further behaviour problems.

Narrative Choices

For an integrative counsellor I have developed an accessible way of using narrative therapy with individual clients. An important discovery from narrative theory is that client problems are often due to narrative clashes between clients and those around them. In Sam's case, he did not see himself as risky, and his mother did not draw attention to the safer parts of his identity. This narrative incoherence plays out by creating escalating interpersonal patterns whereby each person positions the other within their storyline. The technique I use in this situation is called Narrative Choices.

For this approach, the counsellor invites the client to write down all the descriptions they can think of for themselves. Every narrative, every word, including mundane descriptions from shopkeepers and evocative descriptions from ex-partners and school enemies. The words hang separately on the page, disconnected. Figure 8.1a shows an example from Sam's family session.

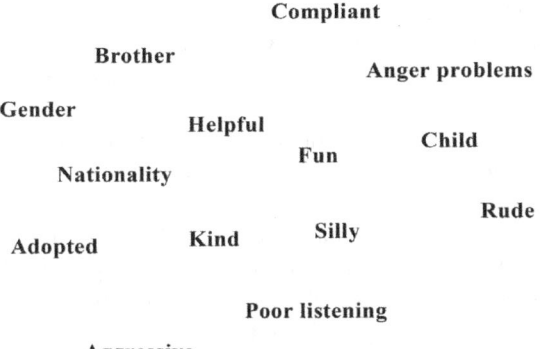

Figure 8.1a Narrative Words

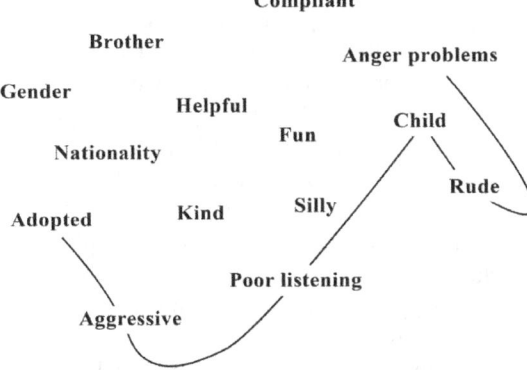

Figure 8.1b The Referral Narrative

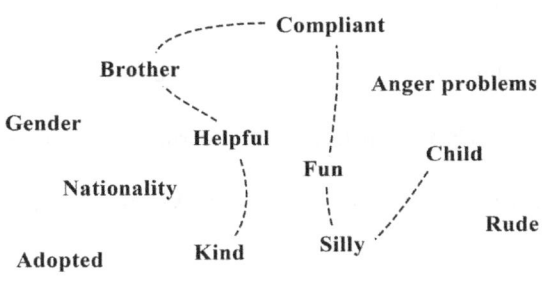

Figure 8.1c The Family Game Narrative

Once the descriptions of the client are on the page, the counsellor asks the client, in coloured pens, to draw connecting lines between words. Each coloured pen refers to a specific perspective on the client. For instance, if we draw the narrative from the referral form, we obtain Figure 8.1b.

Then we stay curious with the client about different narratives. We try and consider as many perspectives as we can on the client. For example, if we drew the narrative that emerged from the family game, we obtain Figure 8.1c.

The narrative choices approach helps clients to make realistic judgements about who they are in different contexts. It gives them space to reflect on their preferred narratives but also not to avoid feedback from others about the problems they experience. The person no longer becomes defined by problem narratives.

Recently I worked with someone in relation to her race identity. She completed the narrative choices activity and noticed how she had lived with narrative incoherence for most of her life. In the context of racism and discrimination, she was narrated in a way that clashed with her sense of self. Often this led to more anger and frustration in trying to escape from these powerful labels. At first, she wrote the words that she had either heard or that had been implied in how she and others describe or narrated her. These were "Loud", "Fun", "Good Friend", "Hardworking", "Unhappy", "Angry", "Passionate", "Caring", "Disruptive", "Ugly", "Self-Centred", "Beautiful", "Uncaring", and "Lacks Motivation".

The client showed a visceral response, one of sadness and one of frustration, that she said resonated with having carried around other people's opinions of her for a long time. She drew a line and connected the words she felt other people most identified with her. These were teachers, family members, and peers who most connected with the words: "Loud", "Unhappy", "Angry", "Disruptive", "Ugly", "Self-Centred", "Uncaring", and "Lacks Motivation".

After this, the client drew a separate connecting line, linking together the words she would describe herself as, and these were the words she most connected with:

"Loud", "Fun", "Good Friend", "Hardworking", "Passionate", "Caring", "Self-Assured", "Beautiful", and "Confident".

The client was visibly moved by seeing the two opposing selves so clearly:

Loud, Unhappy, Angry, Disruptive, Ugly, Self-Centred, Uncaring, and Lacks Motivation.
Loud, Fun, Good Friend, Hardworking, Passionate, Caring, Self-Assured, Beautiful, and Confident.

The client lived the experience of narrative incoherence for many years but had not found a way to articulate it. One of the positive effects of narrative work was in affirming her self-story, and she felt more robust in responding to the way other people positioned her in discourse as a result. In contexts of racism, the sheer number of daily oppressive narratives are incredibly forceful on a client. Michael White and David Epston state clearly that narrative therapy is thus a political action. In seeing the systemic social-constructionist power that racism has on the self of a client, narrative therapy gives people the freedom to explore alternative preferred knowledges of who they are. This can help clients to relive and retell their experiences in ways that are free from the discriminatory gaze. And noticing the effect of separating people from discriminatory narratives led to one of the most famous and useful tools that sprang from the narrative therapy movement.

Externalising: The Problem Is the Problem

Narratives explain why many clients experience psychological problems. In narrative theory, a presenting problem is a sign that a person is living in a negative self-identity saturated with problem narratives. From a narrative perspective, counselling is tricky because it requires a presenting problem and relies mostly on using language to explore that problem. How do we talk about problems without defining the person as the problem? Is it possible to explore the difficulties of a counselling client without amplifying those difficulties for them?

The answer Michael White gives to this question is very interesting. He says that the conversation should attempt to objectify the problem against the practice of objectifying the person. That is, to take the problem to be its own object and to work against the problem as an object in its own right. Often problem narratives take over the client's way of perceiving themselves. Although it looks like self-reflection, paying attention to negative self-images can grow into situations where one struggles to experience anything outside of the problem. White encourages counsellors to see the problem as the problem and not the person. To separate the problem from the person and empower the person against the problem. Separating the problem from the person is called externalising, and it happens in four stages.

Stage 1: Describe the Problem in the Client's Words

In this stage, the counsellor explores problem definitions with the client to gain specific, nuanced understandings of the problem. Using the word "the" acts as a barrier between the client and the problem. What is "the" problem? How big is "it"? What makes "the" problem grow? Where do you usually find "the" problem?

The counsellor is a feedback loop for the client. By encouraging a linguistic separation of the client and the problem, we get to know the client and the problem independently. This positions the client as an observer of the problem and its actions, rather than as being the problem themselves. If we ask someone when "they" feel depressed, or how anxious "they" are, we subtly but powerfully create a sense of self tied up with problem narratives. When people re-story the problem as observers, the linguistic separation can be empowering. What is "the" depression? When is "the" depression strongest? How do you tend to fight off "the" depression? If people live inside stories, then re-storying the problem as the problem is a freeing activity.

Stage 2: Map the Effect of the Problem

The counsellor now has an experience-near definition of the problem. In the second stage, the counsellor and client map the problem's influence and presence in their life, including the client's environment, relationships, feelings, behaviours, aspirations, and thoughts. How does "the" problem affect your relationships? What influence does "the" problem have on your confidence? How is "the" depression affecting your morning routine? What effects is "the" anxiety having on your self-care? By mapping out the problem's effects we learn important details about why the problem is a problem and what the client wants changed.

Stage 3: Evaluate the Effects of the Problem's Activities

In White's externalising approach, the client is encouraged to evaluate the problem's actions and the effects of those actions: Are these activities okay with you? How do you feel about these developments? Is this development positive or negative, or both, or neither, or something in between? We keep an open mind about whether the effects are positive or negative, wanted or unwanted, and we invite the client to speak about their underlying values that oppose the problem. We ask questions like "What do you think about 'the' anxiety making you hyper-focused on people's opinions?" or "Is it a positive or a negative thing that 'the' depression causes you to be on your own at night?" The questions can sometimes sound like leading questions. Questions that are obvious to answer. But clients surprise us in how they evaluate the effects of the problem. Thinking systemically, from a functional point of view, if the narrative has a function, or the problem has a stabilising effect for the client, then the client will counterintuitively figure out that they need the problem in some way. For instance, some clients like that the problem keeps people at arm's-length. Or that the problem prevents them from acting unacceptably. Asking the client to evaluate the effects of the problem requires counsellors to be open-minded about the client's responses.

Stage 4: Justify the Evaluation

In this final step, the counsellor explores the client's orientation towards the evaluation. They are asked why they evaluated the effects as positive or negative. For example, we might ask, "Why is this development good/not good for you?" Justify-the-evaluation questions uncover the value system that underpins the client's social perspective. Clients typically state things like "it's good I'm focused on people's opinions, so I do well in social situations" or "it's bad I'm focused on people's opinions because it makes me shyer in social situations". We can usually predict the type of value system that is evoked, but once the client responds with their rich words, we are led in the direction of their specific social values. In the case where the client likes to focus on opinions, so they do well socially, the underlying reason for liking this effect is that the client values being sociable.

The purpose of these four stages is to separate the problem from the client at the beginning of counselling so that you can support the client against the problem and the problem narrative over the course of the counselling sessions.

Externalising Using Drawing

An approach I have developed with counselling clients, and particularly with children, is externalising using drawing. This approach modifies the original externalising process into a drawing activity.

Stage 1: Draw the problem
Stage 2: Draw the effects of the problem
Stage 3: Evaluate the effects of the problem's activities (draw a + or − for positive/ negative evaluations)
Stage 4: Justify the evaluation with words

One such example comes from a young person working on low mood (see Figure 8.2). He described the problem as a thunderstorm and drew a dark rainy cloud (stage 1). Around the storm were his family members who were scared by the storm, trying to rescue him but without the right tools (stage 2). His emotions were also negatively affected by the storm, and he felt worried, sad, and hopeless (stage 2). He disliked the storm causing worry for his family (stage 3) and drew a red cross beside it. Though the storm created problems for him, he did like that the

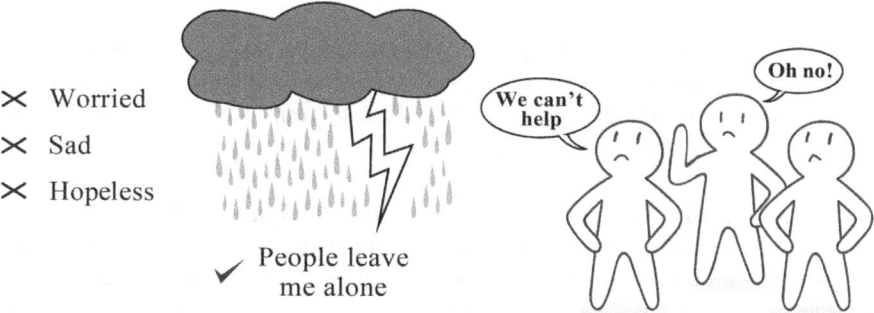

Figure 8.2 Externalised Drawing

storm meant people left him alone (stage 3), and he drew a green tick beside the words "people leave me alone". When asked why he wrote the tick (stage 4), he said because the storm calms down when he has time by himself. He wants to feel calm, and the storm gets stronger if people don't give him space (stage 4).

Externalising separates the client from the problem and begins to uncover resources, hopes, and new narratives. Drawing slows the pace of the session to create a reflective space, and for clients who struggle to externalise, this approach tends to be easier and more accessible.

Unique Outcomes

Clients come to counselling with thick and thin narratives. The more information contained within a self-narrative, the thicker and more real it becomes. Oftentimes, clients benefit from thickening appreciative and affirming narratives. Particularly narratives that have outgrown the problem, and even for a split second.

In his book, *Maps of Narrative Practice*, Michael White adapts the externalising process for focusing on exceptions to the problem, which are unique outcomes that undermine the problem. They often contain solutions the client has been looking for. Thus, drawing attention to unique outcomes can thicken narratives of competence and affirmation. The process runs the same as externalising but with the change or outcome in view:

Stage 1: Describe the unique outcome in the client's words
Stage 2: Map the effects of the unique outcome
Stage 3: Evaluate the effects of the unique outcome
Stage 4: Justify the evaluation

There are a number of reasons to use unique outcomes. Here we return to Sam and his family, from earlier in the chapter, for a final time. Once the family game had come to an end, I decided to verbalise the unique outcomes I had witnessed in the family.

> [Me]: Thank you for completing such a fantastic rollercoaster! Before we finish, I want you to know that I have written down some of the positive differences I saw you make as a family. Before I read them to you, I want you to guess how many positive things I saw [stage 1].

Sam and his family were not sure how to answer the question, but the question seemed to excite their interest. Most families and clients who live in problem narratives barely notice a change when it occurs because they are so habituated to the negative perspective. The idea behind my question was to make the family curious about change, enhance the appreciation the family held of themselves, and thicken narratives against Sam's anger.

After some debate, Sam and his family guessed that I had written down two or three positive things. I asked them to name the possible unique outcomes I had written down (stage 1). They had spotted that Sam was calmer. And that Jess was playing safely. They had also noticed that they had fun together for the first time in a while. I agreed with these observations, and then I told them they were incorrect. Absolutely wrong! In fact, there were 16 positive things written on the page!

The family showed a great deal of surprise at that number, and I asked them to guess one for each family member (stage 1). This line of questioning merges hypothetical questions, which Peter Lang and Elspeth McAdam developed, with appreciative questions, developed by Cooperrider in the late 1990s. To coin a term, they are hypo-appreciative questions that aim at engaging the family's self-appreciation and thickening narratives that counter the problem stories. I attempted to deliver the appreciative feedback in a way that highlighted the circularity of the family's actions. This was to show how individual behaviours are both a response to and a prompt of other family members (stage 2).

I read out loud that Lynn was patient, supportive, and good at listening. This enabled Sam to be good at taking a lead, to show his kindness to his sister, and to feel better (stage 2). This enabled Jess to be fun, to follow instructions, and to be creative (stage 2), which in turn enabled Lynn to show affection, to de-escalate bad moods, and to show support to both children (stage 2).

The family agreed that their play session generated a change in the narratives about each other (stage 2). The family moved from escalation to co-operation, and this reduced the anger and increased the kindness in Sam (stage 2). Lynn said that she was proud to see this change in Sam's anger (stage 3), particularly because she wants him to engage in counselling and be calmer in general (stage 4). Noticing the unique outcomes was resourceful in thickening the family narrative.

The changes in the family were monitored and nurtured over eight weeks of therapy sessions, culminating in a review session where Sam, his mother Lynn, and his sister Jess (with no sign of dad!) rated Sam's anger as no longer an "important" concern for their family. The anger was still creeping in at times, but Sam was free from being defined by it.

Problems, Possibilities, Restraints, and Resources (PPRR)

An effective social-constructionist tool for unpacking pathologising narratives is John Burnham's PPRR quadrant. The tool can be used much more widely than on negative social constructs, but for the purposes of explaining the technique, we will stick to this limited use.

The counsellor or client draws a quadrant on a page with the words "Problems" and "Possibilities" at separate ends of a horizontal line. The words "Restraints" and "Resources" are put at separate ends of an intersecting vertical line, with an empty word bubble in the middle (Figure 8.3). In the centre of the quadrant, the counsellor and client write down a presenting problem, thought, feeling, behaviour, concept,

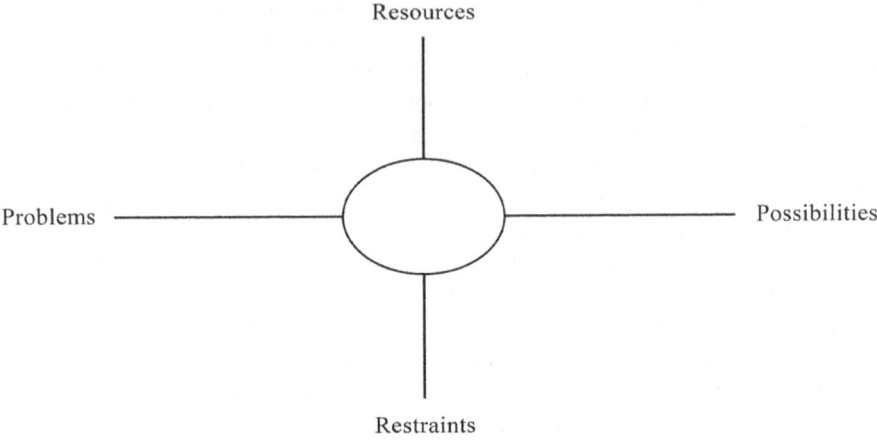

Figure 8.3 PPRR Quadrant

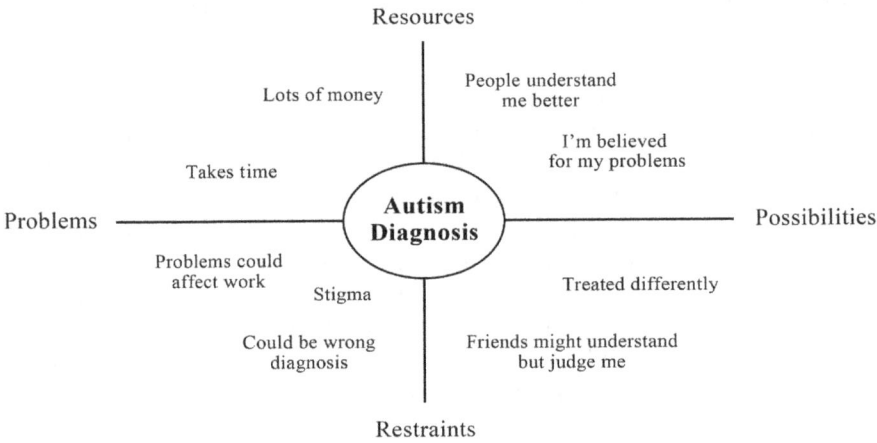

Figure 8.4 PPRR Example

theory, practice, etc., and evaluate it from those four perspectives. The activity is used for seeing the multiple aspects of any counselling phenomenon.

Let's use "autism diagnosis" as a construction to unpack. A counselling client, a 23-year-old male, has said he always felt "different", "weird", and has never "got" implicit social rules that seem natural to his friends. A family member suggested he should investigate an autism diagnosis. He wanted to unpack this in counselling and so we used the PPRR quadrant (see Figure 8.4). When unpacking labels, PPRR encourages questions like, "How could a diagnosis of autism bring about resources in your life?", "Are there ways in which investigating an autism diagnosis might restrain you?", "What possibilities might come out of looking into an autism diagnosis?", "What problems could arise?" Notice the quadrant does not encourage us to think in truth and false terms. Instead, the PPRR model invites counsellors to see any given phenomenon from multiple perspectives.

In this example the client was able to explore whether or not to investigate the diagnosis further and it helped him establish different narratives that complicate the decision. For instance, he wants understanding but not judgement. He wants to be believed for his difficult social experiences but not treated differently. Unpacking the problems and possibilities with diagnosis examined the tensions of an important life decision.

In another case, I have used the quadrant when working with young people who are sectioned under the Mental Health Act with a diagnosis of anorexia nervosa. When meeting one family, for example, we wrote "anorexia" in the central bubble (see Figure 8.5). It might seem counterintuitive to deconstruct the client's presenting problem in this way, but in a systemic view, the problem can be seen as serving some function or being an unhelpful part of the balance in the family. Helping clients unpack the possibilities and resources that their problem affords them can be part of a conversation for finding those resources outside the grip of the problem.

The mother in the family session said that "anorexia" might support the young person in feeling less blamed. This was an interesting statement from the mother. When any culture believes there must be something or someone to blame for a problem, diagnosis absorbs that blame. The disorder can be viewed as outside the person's control. Conversely, the father saw this as a restraint. He said by calling his daughter anorexic we were taking away her responsibility to eat and keep herself alive. He felt his daughter was not disordered but deciding not to eat and saw the importance of accountability. Ignoring the content of these statements for a moment, it is interesting to note that the PPRR activity highlighted a complementary

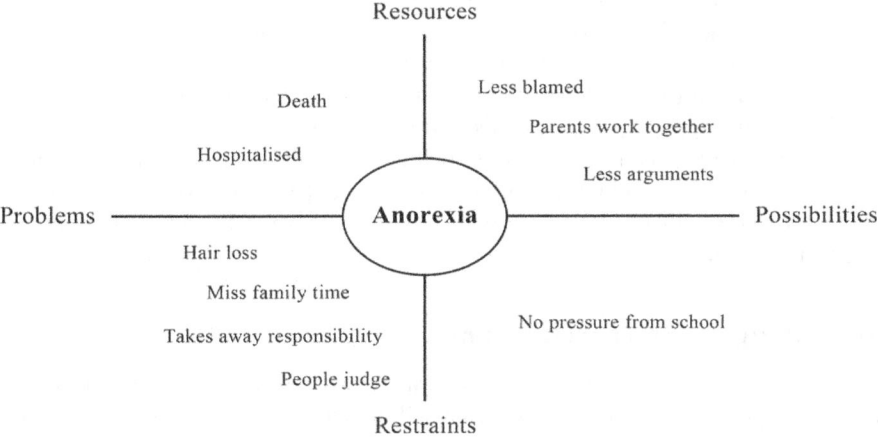

Figure 8.5 PPRR Anorexia

relationship to diagnosis within this family. We revealed something of the pattern of communication within the family simply by deconstructing anorexia.

Burnham developed the PPRR activity further by interviewing families about different positions on the quadrant. We might ask the client a circular question, such as, "when your mother sees the diagnosis as resourceful and your father sees it as restraining, how does this position you?". Viewing different family members or different people in the client's social system as positions on the quadrant draws out relationship patterns and relational insights for how the problem is maintained. It provides the counsellor with a context for some of the issues the client is facing. Melanie Klein, the psychodynamic therapist and researcher, came up with the psychodynamic idea of "splitting", whereby a person cannot tolerate good and bad in things, and so creates a black and white view of reality. Good people and bad people. I am good or I am bad. Klein said that maturity happens when a person realises the inherent goodness and badness in everything. In my experience, Burnham's quadrant has a similar maturing effect on clients. They begin to understand the nuances and complexities of things, being better able to tolerate grey areas.

With an individual client, the counsellor can ask where parents, siblings, partners, managers, and peers would position themselves on the quadrant. For instance, asking, "if your sister was here, what would she say about anorexia?" Or, if we move the issue to depression and suicidality, anxiety and panic, or frustration and anger, "what ways would your friend say this is restraining you? What ways is this giving you a resource?". The PPRR model combines ideas from systems theory, social constructionism, and narrative theory to support clients with reflecting on the way that problems create, inform, affect, and result from interpersonal patterns and social discourse.

Narrative therapy has shown itself to reduce problems related to mental health, for example Lynette Vromans and Robert Schweitzer's work on people with a diagnosis of depression, and it proves its usefulness in work with particular social contexts like gender in the work of Kogeni et al., even when researchers such as Lopes et al. compare narrative with approaches like cognitive behavioural therapy (CBT). Part of the reason for the effectiveness of narrative theory, which the Dulwich Centre and Peter Stratton also attest to, is because it works simultaneously on the mental health problem as well as the social context or construction that brings about the debilitating dominant narrative. By deconstructing meaning, the client perceives themselves differently and often in ways that bring about more hope and understanding.

Counselling Is a Mirrored Room

In this final section of the chapter, we review the work of Hare-Mustin who summarises the learning from narrative counselling with a concept called the mirrored room. What she adds to the discussion so far is in line with second- order cybernetics, which we have described as putting the counsellor into the description of the system. The observer is part of the system.

The mirrored room is the idea that counselling discourse is generated from societal narratives that assert power over clients. Her claim is that "there is a predetermined content in the conversation in therapy" (1994, p. 19) that counsellors have internalised from their surroundings. Hare-Mustin calls for therapists to develop a reflexive awareness to avoid counselling interventions becoming a force for social control.

If language does not simply describe the social world but puts the world into categories, then where do counselling categories come from?

To answer this question, I will discuss a case of externalising. Reminding myself that externalising and narrative therapy were invented to undo debilitating social stories, I was originally baffled as to why the work I am thinking of went horribly wrong.

Here I am thinking of the case of Talia, a 16-year-old young person with whom I tried some narrative and story counselling. I perceived my use of externalising the problem as an ethical intention, a way to separate the anxiety from the client.

Talia's referral was made after she had been diagnosed with generalised anxiety disorder. Hare-Mustin suggests that in accepting a definition of the problem, the counsellor in some way mirrors societal discourses. In Talia's case, she had been displaying fixations, high sensory arousal, and reduced interpersonal communication, consistent with autistic spectrum conditions. I did not explore this because the anxiety hypothesis was successful for the first month in reducing the anxiety for her to return to school. We externalised anxiety and gave it the name "Bob", and this seemed helpful in outmanoeuvring Bob and his negative effects.

Talia's diagnosis and the way I constructed her difficulties may have been influenced by discourses that categorise girls as anxious in a society that encourages girls to internalise problems.

Over a series of weeks, Talia became increasingly isolated, rigid in her behaviours, and, after a violent clash over a sensory issue at home, her mother phoned the police. When Talia's mother asked the police not to enter her room because she has extreme sensory difficulties, the police said that, because Talia was not diagnosed with a sensory difficulty, she remains responsible for her actions, and they entered her room. At this point, Talia lashed out, hit a police officer, and was arrested.

Talia's mother said the period of reduced anxiety followed by a big explosion was a similar pattern to those of previous progresses with other therapists—probably because she is labelled as anxious and not autistic. The anxiety narrative suggests that, with gradual exposure to anxious situations, the problem—"Bob"—reduces. However, what seemed to be happening was that a reduction in the anxiety led to Talia taking part in heightened activity like school, and this new activity overstimulated her, and she withdrew into an anxious ball. This can be seen as a literal example of a dominant discourse becoming a force for social control. In taking on the narrative of anxiety disorder within the counselling sessions, the control of language was partly in my power, perhaps inflaming my unexplored prejudice linking girls with anxiety. This mirrored discourse was borrowed from a professional chain that muted stories about her sensory needs, and for about a decade. Sensory discourses could have stopped her from being arrested and better supported her mother in feeling safe at home. My counselling setting became a mirrored room for stories about anxious girls. And, worryingly, because societal discourse is mirrored in therapeutic settings, a person is twice as likely to receive an autism diagnosis when they are male, even in the situation where the symptoms are identical. In a study by Victoria Milner and colleagues, autistic women reported having felt "different" for a lifetime but understood by others within restrictive stereotypically gendered narratives.

Fred

The mirrored room has drawn attention to the structural inequality in our patterns of working. Taking a second-order position enables counsellors to unpack how their personal and professional stories influence the client. In a more hopeful example, I worked with a young person named Fred. He was 14 years old and referred by his school for scoring highly on a depression scale after his parents divorced. We met up and I asked him about the divorce, which seemed to have no resonance. Was this a defence mechanism? Had he really made his peace with this?

Fred had been through several counsellors with the same persistent low mood. In one of our weekly sessions, I happened to notice that his intonations and voice pitch became overtly masculine, very stereotyped, when discussing girls. It brought up the idea that he was attempting to convince me of his attraction to females. But why? I took the relational risk of asking him about his sexuality. I call this a relational risk, based on the work of Barry Mason, because I come from a context where asking a boy about his sexuality could have been perceived as disrespectful. I wondered about whether counselling had not been safe enough for this conversation due to the surrounding homophobic society.

Fred initially responded by laughing about the question. His increased manly voice, which was quite different from his usual softer tone, became louder. He did not define his sexuality, however, and changed the subject. In my experience, if an issue is not an issue it'll tend to be communicated clearly. "I'm heterosexual". "I genuinely don't care about my parents' divorce". When an issue is an issue, communication becomes muddy. In asking a relationally reflexive question, considering how Fred was experiencing me, a male therapist asking about his sexuality, he said he felt uncomfortable with the question but that he had been questioning his sexuality. Eventually, Fred told me that sexuality had been a untellable discourse for him, particularly among his peers, parents, and supporting professionals, related to his gender and class background, and something he said he felt relieved in discussing with me.

With Fred, I moved to a position of resisting the coercive influence of the mirrored room. Rather than relying on the dominant discourse of the referral, which could have organised me into discussing parental separation, or on my own hesitation about exploring sexuality, I took responsibility for naming and exploring a social grace that appeared organically in the counselling session. It made sense that Fred had requested a new counsellor, more than once. Fred was trying to find a way to talk about being gay. Working out how to navigate his sexuality in a homophobic social environment made up a large proportion of his referral problem. Working on separation might have enhanced my professional knowledge and muted this important emerging story. I drew from similarities in our wider cultural narratives around gender and class in which being gay is constructed as negative, which supported me in addressing the structural inequality in having not addressed sexuality before then.

Fred has since discussed his sexuality with his friends and his mum and said he feels the depression has "nearly gone". One of the milestones in this journey was with his estranged dad having accepted his sexuality as "not a big deal". Fred was certain his dad would not speak with him again, but in changing the discourse in the counselling room, the change carried out into the client's world.

Further Reading

Cooperrider, D. (1999). Positive image, positive action: The affirmative basis of organising. In S. Srivastva & D. Cooperrider (Eds.), *Appreciative management & leadership: The power of positive action and thought in organization* (Rev. ed.) (pp. 91–125). Euclid, OH: Williams Custom Publishing.

Hare-Mustin, R. (1994). Discourses in the mirrored room: A postmodern analysis of therapy. *Family Process, 33*(1), 19–35. doi:1014-7370/93/3301-0019/02.00/0.

Koganei, K., Asaoka, Y., Nishimatsu, Y., & Kito, S. (2021). Women's psychological experiences in a narrative therapy-based group: An analysis of participants' writings and Beck depression inventory–second edition. *Japanese Psychological Research, 63*, 466–475. doi:10.1111/jpr.12326.

Lopes, R., Gonçalves, M., Machado, P. P., & Salgado, J. (2014, November). Narrative therapy vs. Cognitive-behavioural therapy for moderate depression: Empirical evidence from a controlled clinical trial. *Psychotherapy Research, 24*(6), 662–674.

Mason, B. (2005). *Relational risk-taking and the therapeutic relationship in the space between* (pp. 157–170). London: Routledge.

Milner, V., McIntosh, H., Colvert, E., & Happé, F. (2019). A qualitative exploration of the female experience of Autism Spectrum Disorder (ASD). *Journal of Autism and Developmental Disorders, 49*(6), 2389–2402. doi:10.1007/s10803-019-03906-4.

Vromans, L. P., & Schweitzer, R. D. (2011). Narrative therapy for adults with major depressive disorder: Improved symptom and interpersonal outcomes. *Psychotherapy Research, 21*(1), 4–15. doi:10.1080/10503301003591792.

White, M. (2007). *Maps of narrative practice*. London: W. W. Norton & Company.

Chapter 9

Action-Embodiment Counselling

A movement started in the 1800s that pre-emptively charged modern psychotherapies with the crime of (metaphorically) disembodying people from their human
experience. Existentialism, started by the philosopher Kierkegaard, and phenomenology, which came slightly later with the philosopher Husserl, began to examine
the structures of experience as they related to human mortality. The sociologies of
the then-times and the current-times were seen as masking experience through conformity. What people have been taught to experience in a society differs from what
people actually experience. In fact, nearly every intervention in the previous few
chapters, the meaning-making, the contextualising, and the cultural understandings, was named by the founder of gestalt therapy, Fritz Perls, as "mind fucking".

Perls developed the existential-phenomenological position that meaning-making is an intellectual game. It disembodies the client from their experience. He
particularly saw psychoanalysis and other therapies that tried to intellectualise,
rationalise, and analyse client problems as removing people further and further
from their actual felt sense of the world. The metaphor of the system and the cyber-
netic metaphor that underpins much of systems theory leaves little room to even
consider how people experience. In existential terms, society and therapy alike
become forceful repressive powers against a person's authentic experience. We
play interpretive games, like the astrologer, vying for our descriptions to become
experienced by the client as reality. Gestalt therapy says that nobody can claim to
interpret another person's experience. All therapy can do is create the conditions
for genuine experience to emerge.

In this chapter, we describe gestalt techniques using a systemic lens and we
attempt to resolve the sparring match between existential-phenomenological therapies and systemic therapies. Or even to change the game altogether. Is it possible
to integrate phenomenology with systems theory? What would existentialism look
like in the eye of a social constructionist? Would such a project seek to destroy the
foundations of both forms of knowledge?

I don't think so.

DOI: 10.4324/9781003480808-10

Phenomenology and Holism

Holism is the theory that parts of a person are interconnected and cannot exist without reference to the whole person. But experience and behaviour are often fragmented rather than experienced as a whole organism. People have so-called holes in the personality. The word "I" is very important for gestalt therapists because it denotes one experiencing-being. By saying "my" brain doesn't like "the" feelings in "my" stomach, people remove the experiencing "I". A holistic view tries to support the counselling client to fill in the holes in their experience and reclaim disembodied feelings: "I feel sick".

If a person has learned, through fear or coercion, not to show anger, for example, they will disown their anger and project it onto others, never experiencing anger for themselves. Counsellors see the anger by looking at surface behaviours such as the client scratching at their skin or tightening their hands unconsciously around their neck, particularly when discussing an object of their anger, such as a parent, boss, or ex-partner. These subtle acts of turning the anger onto themselves, of doing to themselves that which they cannot do to others, invite the curiosity of the therapist into the client's experience. Phenomenology is the approach that invites all the client's experiences without making interpretations. These experiences range from thoughts to perceptions, from memories to fantasies, from emotions to desires, and from awareness of the body to awareness of the language, meanings, and voice tones that one expresses.

When a person repeatedly projects their experience outwards, or introjects values and judgements from society inwards, they split off their existence and become disorganised and mentally unwell. The idea here is that people need to be whole people, not fake automatons of society, to function as healthy citizens. Fritz Perls and the psychologists before him called the integration of projected parts of the self a "Gestalt," which is the German word for "organised whole". It is our ability to experience our authentic selves against the distortions that occur when we defend against uncomfortable and distressing feelings.

Phenomenological Inquiry

A counsellor using a gestalt approach switches questions of why with questions of how. Instead of "why do you experience your sadness?", which invites a meaning-making intellectual task, ask "how do you experience your sadness?". Probing the client's experience is named phenomenological inquiry because the counsellor tries to bring awareness to the experiential component of a memory or an emotion, or any phenomenon in experience. Above interpretation and ideas, experience is the highest authority.

The important orientation here is to ask questions about the here-and-now moment-to-moment experience of the client. An example comes from a client recently having separated from her boyfriend. The client said she was annoyed because her boyfriend spread rumours that made her appear like a terrible person. Their shared friendship group stopped speaking with her. She said she was annoyed "because" he was victim-blaming her to avoid his own guilt of having cheated in the relationship. She proceeded to provide one example after another to support this interpretation. The word "because" here, to a counsellor interested in phenomenology, indicates that the client is moving from her current experience to ideas in her head. This rationalisation takes clients out of being aware of the experience, often into repetitive rationalisations that merely compound emotional detachment. Many counsellors struggle with the broken-record nature of a client frustratedly, and sometimes monotonously, circling around a point without taking a breath. Wanting to use phenomenological inquiry, I asked my client to describe her tone of voice. This small but crucial activity of phenomenology switches from explaining the experience to describing the experience. Doing so activates the current experience and emotions begin to surface.

The client said her voice was "annoyed". In a heartbeat, she quickly said "because" her ex-boyfriend was a victim-blamer in his previous relationship. Again, the client runs the risk of explaining, of using interpretation and becoming separated from her experience. I asked if she could describe her voice, how was it showing annoyance? She said her voice was quick, loud, and she could feel her throat tightening up. As she became aware of her annoyance, she began to cry. She said it's like there's a little child inside her trying to tell her to hide.

The "why" question would take away the tears. The experience would possibly disappear into a broken-record barrage of explanations. Instead, using phenomenology, I asked how she experiences this little child. In the present moment, what experience is she having? She said she feels a deep sadness and fear. I asked her to speak from the perspective of the child, in the here-and-now. She said, "nothing ever goes my way" and she began to cry further. She said, "no-one ever takes my side. Everyone always turns against me".

These words were brighter, more visceral. She was contacting a forming-gestalt. Part of her experience was coming through. Her authentic experience was that nobody stays on her side.

Figure-Ground

In gestalt psychotherapy, Fritz Perls and his colleagues used knowledge from experimental psychology to show how people experience the world by focusing on some aspects and neglecting others. The classic example is the face-vase, whereby looking at the face makes the vase vanish, and looking at the vase overlooks the face (Figure 9.1).

Holism or gestalt formation is the recognition that this picture is both a vase and a face. Or, analogously, if we experience no one as on our side, we overlook those who are. Perls and his colleagues used the idea of holism to describe how figures we see in the foreground of our experience show what we are primed to focus on. We experience our environment only in parts and place many things, such as our anger, our sadness, and our worry into the background. Why do some people see faces first? Others vases? Why do some people experience worlds where everyone is on their side or where no one is on their side?

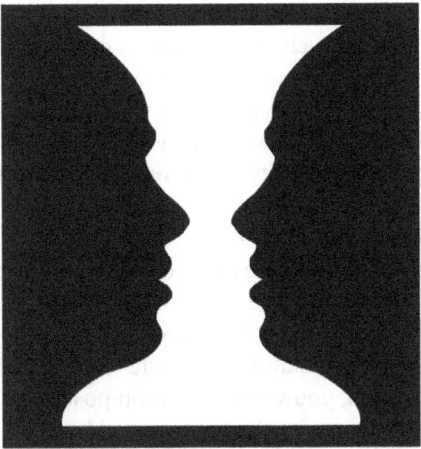

Figure 9.1 Face-Vase

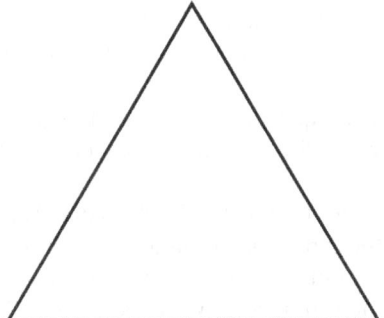

Figure 9.2 Triangle Perspective

Figure 9.2 depicts a triangle. An exercise to understand the figure-ground relationship is to consider different sides of the triangle as the base. For example, changing the base in your mind from the bottom line to the line on the left. Try it. With your imagination, imagine the triangle is on its side, or upside down. That different points of the triangle, different sides, are the bottom. You should perceive the triangle change.

Had you not been invited to change your perspective on the triangle, your perspective would likely have been fixed on the perceived fact that the triangle is standing upright. The base is at the lowest point. This is similar to the situation when a person has acquired defence mechanisms, and when people defend against their experience. Their experience organises their perceptions into fixed gestalts. These are unresolved situations where the client has not grown. Imagine a fixed gestalt as a situation where you see all triangles in a particular orientation. Now transpose the triangle for an emotion or social role such as authority. When people who have unfinished business with authority come to counselling, they will usually find ways to evoke the punishing authority of the counsellor. Their perception co-creates the counsellor's authoritative reaction if the counsellor is not careful. This is to say that if a person has learned to experience authority as abusive, and has not resolved this, they will also experience the counsellor's authority as abusive.

In gestalt language, the client has "unfinished business" when they fixate on certain ways of experiencing without taking in other perspectives or other possible experiences. The theory is that the client will experience the world through the prism of "nobody is on my side" when they have learned this fixed gestalt or pattern of experience. A common example of a fixed gestalt is times where you need to post a letter or a birthday card. In this situation, you will focus in on postboxes, and, suddenly, they seem to be everywhere, in places you had not noticed before— they were in the background and are now in the foreground. If you turn 30, you see marriage everywhere. If you hurt your finger, you become painfully aware of that finger's role in every basic task. These figures of experience reveal something about us as people in our current mode of experiencing. By focusing on what the clients' figures are, at the obvious level, we access their unfinished business, how they discriminate one image from another in their environment. The things that limit their growth.

Systems theory comes into view by considering questions like how do people develop unfinished business? Why do some people focus on the glass being half full and others on the glass being half empty?

The answer to these questions, given by Bateson earlier in this book, is that from experience people learn contexts and patterns for experiencing. In gestalt therapy, as in systems theory, people interpret the world through patterns they have developed from childhood, adolescence, adulthood, and from society. As Perls himself said, it becomes easy to find and live by a pattern rather than by awareness and observation. Living by awareness and observation is a gestalt, the ability to be present in our experience in the moment. It brings up questions like, "How much of our social contact do we spend on autopilot?", "How much are we tuned in dynamically with the situation, not using our ready-made interpretations and responses?". In most of this book, systems theory is offering something to another counselling approach. In this case, systems theory is taking from gestalt theory that people tend to become fixed on unique patterns of experiencing. Probing into that experience is an important step in discovering (and escaping from) aspects of their world.

For human beings, patterning is unavoidable and desirable. The point is not to eradicate the patterns by which we interpret the world but to observe and become aware of those patterns, those organised ways of living, which trap us in psychological distress. Changing the pattern is possible by doing something different, but if people respond to our difference by positioning us into old patterns or old stories then we find our way back into the pattern. How many times have you tried not to argue with someone, or tried not to enter a pattern of procrastination, only to find yourself invited by your antagonist or environment into behaving in the old way? Perls would say that observation and awareness bring about a gestalt, and systemic therapists agree with this. It is simply that we see how this change leads to effects in our environment which form part of a fuller gestalt, an ecology of patterning. Bateson calls this an ecology of mind because the world forms part of our experience and our experience forms part of the world.

The Empty Chair

It is not possible to talk about gestalt therapy without mentioning the famous and incredibly effective gestalt technique, the empty chair (Figure 9.3). The client is invited to explore conflicts, gestalt formations, experiences, and unfinished business, moving between two chairs—a chair which they occupy and an empty chair. To help the client increase their awareness of aspects of their experience, the counsellor encourages the client to embody content from the session, to play the role of the content, in the empty chair.

Let's imagine a client speaking in whispers when they tell you about the rejection they faced in the workplace. We use phenomenological inquiry to ask the client to describe their voice. The feeling and tenor of their voice is described as low in confidence. As the counsellor, you invite the client to put the low confidence in the empty chair. As "low confidence", the client is encouraged to speak in the here-and-now and to create a dialogue.

As "low confidence" the client begins, rather nastily, to scold the client. Low confidence says things like "You are not worth anything" and "Why would your colleagues even want to talk to you?". We notice, and this is crucial, that the "low confidence" character is very confident indeed, much louder and more self-assured

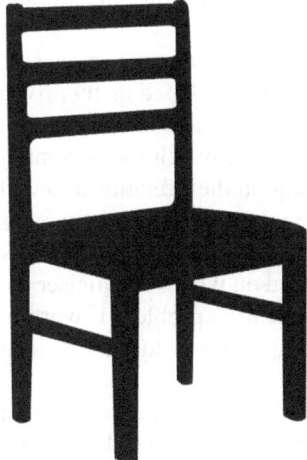

Figure 9.3 Empty Chair

than the client. And more direct. When we invite the client to respond, shyly, she says, "I don't want you to say things like that to me". And, importantly, the client stops responding. She freezes. Now we invite "low confidence" to respond. The client animates, becomes bigger and louder, "See, you can't even say anything. You've got nothing to say! I'm here to protect you. You can't even talk properly!".

When the client returns to her seat, she has discovered something. Not that she is fundamentally unconfident, but that her lack of confidence protects her from facing social rejection. The idea of the empty chair is that the client becomes more aware and understanding of their emotions and of their needs by experiencing several aspects of themselves in the empty chair. This is not a process of interpretation but a process of self-discovery. The client identified more with the critical part of herself, and low confidence resulted. Over time, the client was able to challenge low confidence, give it advice, tell it she does not need protecting. It is important to remember that she is talking to herself. Many clients come out of the activity feeling emboldened, as though they have talked with someone or something real. What is real, if the counsellor keeps their presence to a minimum, is that the client begins to experience themselves, fully. Even where awful abuses have occurred, it is the person's organism that carries that abuse forward, using self-defeating behaviours to mask unfinished, unprocessed, unconscious trauma. Using the empty chair, the client expresses feelings that were previously interrupted with intellectualisations. As a result, her needs and emotions came to life.

The Monodrama

In the empty chair technique, by concerning ourselves with the visceral truth of a client's presenting problem, we lose the circularity of their interaction patterns. A systemic rendition of the empty chair technique is called monodrama, which gives language to a client's embodied knowledge as well as their meaning-making and interpersonal interactions.

In the monodrama, the client plays a variety of roles, and is the only person, so to speak, on stage. My example here comes from work I have developed in my private clinic and can be thought of as one of a plethora of expressions of a monodrama. In my approach, the client thinks of someone or somewhere in which the presenting problem is visible. In this example, the client is working on their relationship with being criticised. The client selects three or four participants (friends, family members, teachers, colleagues) and labels chairs (or assigns the chairs without labels) to represent the different people. Selection happens based on who is a criticiser and who is a supporter of the client. This is because the presenting problem is working on responding to criticism. Had the problem been eating issues or low self-esteem then the people would have been relevant to those problems.

Once the characters in the monodrama are established, the client moves between the chairs as directed by the counsellor. With the client in chair one, the client is invited to explain to the criticiser the impact and experience of their criticism. Our client, who is a female in her early twenties struggling with anxiety around criticism, begins to explain how the judgemental comments from her dad, particularly around her weight and her intelligence, have caused her to withdraw from him and hate herself. Immediately, she begins to get in touch with the emotion of the criticism from her dad. She begins to cry. I encourage her to continue to speak to the criticiser, to the imagined critical father, and she says, "You think it's funny, but it really hurts". And her emotions continue to pour out.

Then, I encourage the client into the chair of the critical-other and for a dialogue to develop. As her critical father, she shares a different perspective. He says that as her father he is only trying to bond with her. He doesn't mean to be hurtful. He is sad to hear how the comments affect her but thinks she is taking them too seriously. Shifting the client back into her seat, she says she can recognise his intention but, in reality, he is horrible, and his jokes are hurtful.

A phenomenological-systemic inquiry is possible, sticking with the two chairs. As in, we could continue to build on this interpersonal pattern in terms of the client's experience of their relationship with their father. But a new route is opened in the monodrama. By asking the client to take up one of the supporter chairs, the client embodies different perspectives and emotional vantage points in her relationship system. In this situation, the client chooses her boyfriend. He, ignoring the father, tells the client how great she is as a person and how her dad is just insecure himself. The client, seeming more emboldened, responds, as herself, and agrees with the boyfriend. She says she knows her father is insecure but still struggles with his comments. Then, a second supporter is invited into the conversation. This time, the client chooses her mother. Her mother speaks directly to the father, with a louder voice, being assertive. The mother tells the father to stop the hurtful comments. She reprimands him for putting their daughter down. The new system has a more empowered feel to it.

The young person, playing all these roles herself, was revealing a complex web of interpersonal patterns. The triangulation between her, her mother, and her father, was important to the way she responded to criticism and to how the father engaged with his daughter. Her increase in self-esteem when internalising her boyfriend's comments and her increase in assertiveness when playing her internalised mother were important resources to draw on, as well as exploring how these supportive positions take an "anti-dad" tone and influence the pattern between them. The monodrama revealed a variety of lifecycle issues, circular causations of anxiety, systemic criticism (of daughter and father), familial disputes, social developments about image conscientiousness, and all within an action-embodied piece of individual "therapy theatre". At the end of the monodrama, the client becomes themself again and reflects on the process.

Enactment

The monodrama relies on working with the internalised systems of individual clients. Sometimes counsellors have the privilege of having real systems in the room. The monodrama and empty chair techniques are like a systemic technique called "enactment" in which multiple clients are asked to speak with each other rather than to the counsellor. We invite clients, sometimes a family, a subsystem of a family, or a couple, to re-enact a difficult conversation from the last week. Something where the presenting problem is present. In the original iteration of enactment, developed by Salvador Minuchin, the counsellor withdraws from the conversation to become an observer while the family, or a subset of the family, holds a meaningful discussion.

The technique is enormously generative. Within the first few interactions, a pattern is revealed. This is provided that the counsellor pays close attention to the process and not the content of the discussion. Drawing on the circumplex model, which reflects on how flexible, bonded, and communicable the family is, an enactment reveals the family's process for constructing flexibility/rigidity, cohesion/distance, and communication. When clients describe their interactions, they often have not seen or experienced the facts of their interpersonal patterns relationally.

This actively embodied technique can be adapted for individuals, using a quasi-empty-chair approach. The counsellor invites an interaction between a client and their system, be it a friendship group, a work relationship, a family, or some other important relationship. In moving between the different positions, the counsellor can unpack interactions and meanings that are being created. There is also room for probing into the embodied experiences of the interaction sequence. Seeing the system in flow is a valuable resource in understanding presenting problems.

Psychodrama

Enactment, monodrama, and the empty chair technique belong to a long history of dramatic counselling methods that the psychiatrist Jacob Moreno pioneered in the early 1920s. Moreno was experimenting with therapeutic theatre, and discovered that using action methods, in which people role-play emotional situations, anxiety-provoking conflicts, and hopeful interactions, people benefit psychologically when returning back to their lives. Using drama as a psychological tool, which is the basic principle of psychodrama, provides different counselling options for people who benefit from movement, action, and embodiment. Much of the talking cure, as far as it emphasises linguistic forms of expression, is restricted by the many years of psychological defences that hijack the language faculty to avoid being present in experiences and emotions.

The notion of "action techniques" sprang from the psychodrama movement, inspiring creative confrontative techniques in the systemic and gestalt field. Moreno maintained that drama was a meaningful way to explore the truth of someone's experience and the social roles people take on. In combining phenomenology, which focuses on the structure of experience, with systems theory, which emphasises social interactions, Moreno grounded psychodrama in the principle that through taking on roles in drama, people gain new perspectives, new skills, new emotional thresholds, for moving beyond their current state of awareness and psychological capacity. It is not so much acting as developing the self by means of re-acting.

One problem that people face is that by reacting in real situations they have suddenly defined a social relationship. People sit on the precipice of deciding to express frustration or depression to a loved one, or to challenge a bullying authority figure. The safety and make-believe of psychodrama gives people a chance to repeat, create, and practise ways of responding to life situations without the burden of concretising their social relations. In real life, the more roles we play free from conflict, the healthier we become. Psychodrama gives clients a way to rehearse and improvise who they are in each context. The practices that grow from an action-embodiment form of counselling are always trying to enrich, brighten, and contact experience with an eye towards the relationships and systems that are created. Moreno discusses the importance of learning to trust the body of the client by using action. Hearing, seeing, and sensing the world through their eyes and ears, using action techniques, engages clients with authenticity and understanding.

Dream Work

Action and embodiment counselling integrates systems theory with the philosophy of experience. It homes in on individual dynamics and pulls back to consider the system dynamics that are impacted by individual changes. The individual grows in relation to their environment and the environment changes in relation to the individual. Fritz Perls was well aware of this connection because one of the key theories underpinning gestalt therapy is field theory. This theory, developed by Kurt Lewin, states that a person's behaviour is a function of their environment. Field theory stresses individual responsibility and growth; systems theory stresses relational responsibility and social growth. Using both lenses to examine client problems is resourceful for counsellors.

The integration of these ideas is clear when working with dreams. Fritz Perls used a powerful, action-embodiment technique in which a person retells a memorable, recurrent dream or nightmare. Perhaps a better description is that the client relives the dream or nightmare in the present moment. Perls described a dream as an existential message. A message about a person's existence, their way of experiencing, and a message that can be deciphered by the gestalt process.

An example comes from a young woman who came to counselling following separation anxiety when leaving her parents' home for work. When alone, she found herself suddenly taken by panic attacks, questioning her health, and feeling an urge to return home. She began to have nightmares that would wake her up in fits of anxiety.

In dream work, we support the client to find the existential message from the dream. First, we ask the client to tell us the dream. After the details are clear, we encourage the client to position themselves as a stage director, to set the stage for the dream by talking in the present tense, as though the dream is happening now. When important parts of the dream arise, signalled by heightened emotion, withdrawal, or some phenomenon like a tapping foot, the counsellor invites the client to take on the role of those parts, to bring them to life. The client is encouraged to play the component parts of the dream. For instance, the client plays the role of a person or object in the dream. They might become their tapping foot or their strangling hands. Once the components of the dream are worked on, the client begins to make sense of the dream. They tend to learn something from within the dream about their experience. Something previously hidden.

In the case of our client, we worked on a nightmare:

> I am driving down the street in my car and hear some people shouting at me. I get really scared. No matter how fast I try to drive away, they catch up and get hold of me, pulling me out of the car. One of the people has a plank of wood and jumps off his bike, coming towards me. I am frightened but cannot move. He looks evil and keeps coming towards me. I am feeling paralysed. He hits the piece of wood against the lamppost with such force that it creates an enormous sound that shrieks into my ears. The sound creates so much fear in me that I wake up.

In dramatising this nightmare, the client was invited into the role of the shrieking sound. The sound made statements about being unsafe and uncertain, "I'm coming but you don't know what I am". She was asked to play the role of the person with the plank of wood, of the frozen girl (herself), of the car, and so on. The client immediately began to make surprising connections to real-life events. One memory came back, something she had not thought about for many years. She was a child in a new school, alone for the first time after her mum had dropped her off, and some students chased her into an empty classroom with sticks in their hands and hit her with them. She was paralysed with fear. The other memory was of being in her bedroom and hearing a frightening slap sound, which she believed was her father hitting her mother in the next room. Again, she was paralysed with fear. She did not know what had happened to her mum or what might happen to her if she made a sound. The sound of the wood hitting the lamppost in the dream was the same sound as the father hitting her mother in real life.

In both cases the message was, when you are alone, away from mum, you are not safe. This was her existential message. In both cases she became clingier to her mum. From a gestalt perspective the client became aware of her fear of separation. She assimilated that fear by connecting it with events in her life. And crucially she disowned part of the message about being unsafe on her own, because she is now a capable adult, gaining success in her life.

There is nothing here from a systemic perspective that is clashing. The client is simultaneously working on her fragmented personality because her system of interpretations has changed from an unprocessed state of "I am unsafe when alone" to a processed state of "I can be safe when I'm alone". Systems theory was not designed to describe the components of a dream and of a person's personality, or of someone's experience, but this is not problematic for integrating these ideas.

Another way of seeing the same information is that the client has reframed what it is like to be alone. Now the systemic counsellor considers how the client's new awareness could affect her and her relationship with her mum, because the unsafety she experienced may have been serving some interpersonal function.

The client's panic attacks went, and she got to the point where she started to work on buying her own home with her partner. Her mother showed a hurtful lack of curiosity towards her new relationship, and this caused some issues between them. The feedback loop of her reduction in anxiety was met with more anxiety-provoking responses—as if, non-consciously, to keep the system as it was. Working on the life cycle of moving on from home was important to allow her new character to gain footing in this family and social life. Integratively, we took some of the power out of the client's dream and gave it back to her. We helped her integrate her own existential dilemma, that of being unsafe when alone, to take on more responsibility and find her own safety. But we keep our eyes on the systemic effects of the change and use the double-lens to know which interventions to draw on and move forward with. When the client finished the counselling, moving between the two lenses was significant in her remaining stable in her family position and personal development.

The Not-Knowing Position

Systems approaches and experiential approaches have in common that a curiosity to learn about the client's reality is a founding principle of counselling. Harlene Anderson and Harold Goolishian, two collaborating psychologists, named this as the client being the expert about their own life. The systems theorist sees the client's interactional patterns and meanings as one kind of expertise. The phenomenological theorist sees the client's experience as a second kind of expertise. Anderson and Goolishian argued against the separation of systemic knowledge and existential knowledge. As a result, they developed the concept of the not-knowing position, in which counsellors situate themselves as curious explorers within the client's reality.

The counsellor is encouraged to hold on to their professional knowledge. For example, the knowledge that people expand their consciousness by becoming aware of dimmed, hidden, or denied experiences. But this nomothetic knowledge, which means their general knowledge, should be translated by the client's words, behaviours, and experiences into specific knowledge of the client. We do not interpret their world for them. The person knows everything, and we are in a position of not knowing. We must find out what their world consists of. When a client brings forward their experience, we may fit it together into a discovery. For instance, when a client uncovers the message from her nightmare, "You are unsafe when alone", and she tells us about two linked memories, we help her to organise her experience into a narrative.

Using the not-knowing position means being alert to the language and responses of the client. Phenomenologically, we probe into feelings, use drama to play out

dreams, and highlight body language. Systemically, we probe into interaction patterns, verbal and gestural meanings, and dominant narratives. In each case we are
trying to do so from a position of not knowing. Fritz Perls said that any interpretation is a therapeutic mistake. It interferes with the client's self-discovery. By taking
a not-knowing stance, the counsellor shows openness to what the client says and
feels.

The Internalised Other Interview

A good way of thinking about not knowing is by inviting clients to sit imagina-
tively in the realities of the people around them. An action-embodiment technique
is not required to be about the client's personal experience. It can be about the client's experience of another person's experience. One technique, pioneered by Karl
Tomm, was developed to allow clients to enter the world of other people in their
relationship systems. It is called the "internalised other interview" or "IOI" for
short. This dramatic technique, in keeping with John Burnham's clarification of the
steps, starts by selecting a person for the client to role-play. For example, a client
might play a parent, one of their children, a sibling, one of their friends, or a work
manager. The counsellor discusses how the IOI can connect with the goal of the
interview. For example, a person working on assertiveness might find it useful to
enter into their manager's perspective. Particularly if they have internalised a manager under which showing assertiveness is impossible. The client is then grounded
in the identity of the other by asking them their name, age, and where they work.
Grounding questions should be relevant to the selected person and in psychodrama
they enable clients to immerse themselves into the role of the selected character.

Once the client is grounded in the identity of their selected person, the IOI
explores the experience of the other with reference to the interview goals. Working
with assertiveness, we might ask the manager, "What have you noticed about the
client's level of assertiveness?". This can draw out the internalised sense of self
from the client. We may consider ways of bringing out internalised values, for
example, "What are your beliefs on workers being assertive towards you as the
manager?" or we may ask for distinctions like "What is the difference between
hostility and assertiveness?". To explore the internalised resources of the manager,
perhaps for the client to borrow in their life outside of the counselling room, we
might ask, "What makes you assertive? How did you develop your assertiveness?".
The idea is to unpack the internalised manager, brother, or friend, to consider what
the client is responding to in their lack of assertiveness. This is true of any goal.
For instance, if we were exploring depression or anxiety, the interview would focus
on how the internalised person, by being internalised, is influential towards the
presenting problem in the client, positively or negatively.

After this, the deeper experience of the selected character is explored. The IOI
explores the relationship between them and the client. Circular and reflexive questions bring about distinctions of importance. For instance, "When the client is nervous around you, how does this position you?". Or we might explore desires and

hopes such as "If the client was more assertive at work, what positive changes might this bring about?". After the internalised other has explored their relationship with the client, then the interview ends, and the two characters are encouraged to de-role and say their goodbyes. At this point, the counsellor and client reflect on the IOI process and the effects it is having on the client's relationship to the presenting problem.

Double Description

In existentialism and systems theory there is no ultimate meaning to a person's experience. Systemic counsellors describe patterns and narratives rather than providing ultimate explanations for the patterns. Valid perspectives are endless. The early gestalt psychologists were seen as part of the systemic movement by Gregory Bateson. Early in this book we noted the gestalt outlook, that if you see in three dimensions, it is because you take information with one eye and another eye to create more depth about what you are seeing. The counselling eye on the situation creates more depth from joining different perceptions. Such a double description is a way to add depth to a person's experience and vision of their relationship.

Gestalt psychologists connect the perceptual field to the innate needs of the person. For instance, a person who has the need to feel accepted and who grows up in a sporty environment might attach social acceptance with doing well in sports. Or a person who grows up in a liberal environment might attach social acceptance with political positions like being environmentally friendly and pro social change. When something enters the perception of either of these two people, their way of seeing the object will depend on how the object connects or not to their needs. A person's description and perception are tied up with their needs. If something meets a person's needs, it becomes foregrounded or brought into awareness. If something does not meet a person's needs, it becomes backgrounded or pushed out of awareness. Phenomenology is saying that people select things to focus on, to be aware of, based on some interconnection with their physical, social, and emotional needs. Systems theory simply adds that the individual is part of maintaining balance in their environment and so how people perceive links also with what is good for their relationships, even if bad for their individual needs.

Action techniques bring forward emotional, cognitive, imaginative, behavioural, and interpersonal experience, bridging the gap between experience and meaning with double descriptions of client realities and problems. Counsellors need not separate different forms of experience, brought forward through the narrowing limits of our modalities. We can choose to develop a technique in the direction of personal growth or circular insight, simply by adding more descriptions and more perspectives on to the situation with the client.

Sculpting

Action and embodiment techniques are shortcuts for observing meaning and experience in action. Family therapy uses sculpting as an active-embodiment technique to uncover meaning and experiences of family members. In sculpting, the counsellor invites a family member to arrange the family into a static sculpture that represents their experience as a family member. The counsellor asks questions about space, posture, positioning, proximity. Are people standing? Who is close by? How do the faces look? Sad? Happy? Frustrated? As the family member completes the sculpture, the others are asked to be passive participants, being shaped by the requests of where to sit, stand, and how. When the person has created their sculpture, they take a position within it.

An example of a male client with depression was that he positioned his mother, father, and sister, all together in a line, smiling, looking out at the sun through the window. He, on the other hand, was very much in the back of the room, metres away, alone in the darkened corner. I interviewed the family members about their experience within the sculpture. The father became upset, saying he felt he was closer to his son than his son had shown. Being quiet, and being withdrawn, had meant the client had not made his experience within the family known. The sculpture visualised the client's experience of depression. I then asked him to sculpt the family in a way that would reduce the depression. He went over and met his family halfway, positioning his sister as hugging him and inviting him into the sunnier side of the room. Having inquired about the phenomenology of the sculpture, in terms of the felt experience, we then explored the meaning from the client's point of view. For him, this voiced a hidden experience: the family seemed happy without him.

With individual clients, sculpting is possible using objects and drawings. For example, scrunched up pieces of paper can represent different family members and so can objects like toy figures. The purpose is to find ways to access the multiplicity of meanings and experiences that clients bring to counselling. Action therapy is co-constructed by the client and counsellor. To be inclusive of difference, we should avoid privileging one form of meaning-making. Experiences, memories, hopes, traumas, losses, and fears are embodied as well as analysed and remembered. They are not only accessed through language. Sculpting explores problems physically and sensorily rather than relying on words or explanations.

The literature on mind-body-meaning connections in counselling shows a reduction in many of the presenting problems in clients. For example, Williams et al. showed that mindful approaches reduce depression, and Staples et al. found the same result when adding systemic techniques such as genograms. Smeeding et al.'s research on anxiety discovered similar findings, that tuning into the body through breathing or action techniques reduces worry and concern, with Moodley et al. finding that a systemic and cultural dimension to the therapy assists outcomes when it affirms cultural realities. The techniques in this section serve as momentary guides in an ever-growing relationship between action, embodiment, and systems theory. In the final chapter we attempt to bring the learning acquired so far in the book together in one place, considering how and why to move from embodied experience and action to different modalities within a systemic integrative framework.

Further Reading

Anderson, H., & Goolishian, H. (1992). The client is the expert: A not-knowing approach to therapy. In S. McNamee & K. J. Gergen (Eds.), *Therapy as social construction* (pp. 25–39). London: Sage Publications, Inc.

Burnham, J. (2000). Internalized other interviewing: Evaluating and enhancing empathy. *Clinical Psychology Forum, 140*, 16–20.

Husserl, E. (1989). *Ideas pertaining to a pure phenomenology and to a phenomenological philosophy*. Boston: Springer.

Kierkegaard, S. (1959). *Either/or*. New York: Doubleday.

Lewin, K. (2008). *Resolving social conflicts and field theory in social science*. Washington, DC: American Psychological Association.

Minuchin, S., & Nichols, M. P. (1993). *Family healing Tales of hope and renewal from family therapy*. New York: Free Press.Moodley, R., Sutherland, P., & Oulanova, O. (2008). Traditional healing, the body and mind in psychotherapy. *Counseling Psychology Quarterly, 21*(2), 153–165. doi:10.1080/09515070802066870.

Moreno, J. L. (1946). *Psychodrama* (1st vols). Beacon House. doi:10.1037/11506-000.

Moreno, J. L. (1994). *Psychodrama since moreno* (M. Karp & M. Watson, Eds.). London: Routledge.

Nichols, M. P., & Fellenberg, S. (2000). The effective use of enactments in family therapy: A discovery-orientated process study. *Journal of Marital and Family Therapy, 26*, 143–152.

Papp, P., Scheinkman, M., & Malpas, J. (2013). Breaking the mould: Sculpting impasses in couples' therapy. *Family Process, 52*, 33–45.

Perls, F. (1969). *Ego, hunger, and aggression; The beginning of gestalt therapy*. New York: Random House.

Perls, F., Hefferline, R., & Goodman, P. (1951). *Gestalt therapy: Excitement and growth in the human personality*. New York: Dell.

Smeeding, S. J., Bradshaw, D. H., Kumpfer, K., Trevithick, S., & Stoddard, G. J. (2010). Outcome evaluation of the veterans affairs salt lake city integrative health clinic for chronic pain and stress-related depression, anxiety, and post-traumatic stress disorder. *Journal of Alternative & Complementary Medicine, 16*(8), 823–835.

Staples, J., Atti, J., & Gordon, J. (2011). Mind-body skills groups for posttraumatic stress disorder and depression symptoms in Palestinian children and adolescents in Gaza. *International Journal of Stress Management, 18*(2), 246–262. doi:10.1037/a0024015.

Starr, A. (1977). *Rehearsal for living: Psychodrama*. Chicago: Nelson Hall.

Tomm, K. (1987b). Interventive interviewing: Part II. Reflexive questioning as a means to enable self-healing. *Family Process, 26*, 153–183. doi:10.1111/j.1545-5300.1987.00167.

Williams, M., Teasdale, J., Segal, Z., & Kabat-Zinn, J. (2007). *The mindful way through depression: Freeing yourself from chronic unhappiness*. New York: The Guilford Press.

Chapter 10

Systemic Integrative Counselling

This book has presented a model called Systemic Integrative Counselling, or "SIC" for short, which underscores the most common counselling modalities with a systemic perspective. In this final chapter, we summarise the main parts of SIC and describe the model in full. SIC is premised on the idea that the obligation to choose between counselling models is a false one. Each model describes and articulates aspects of the client's reality, even if presenting as a fundamental truth. The dimensions of a client's problem get lost inside the narrowness of counselling models, and stepping into other approaches, integrating between counsellor-descriptions of client problems, broadens the therapeutic horizon. My intention is not to present a fully integrated psychotherapy. I do not think this is possible. The point is to find something new.

It has been possible to integrate counselling modalities with a systemic framework by drawing on the efforts of John Burnham and the Approach-Method-Technique (AMT) Model. In AMT, counselling techniques can be moved from one modality into a systemic theory or approach when the counselling technique is used in a circular way. The AMT model says that a counselling theory or approach creates methods or ways of working that inspire particular techniques and interventions. If we are consistent with our theory, we can integrate interventions or techniques from one modality to another by re-theorising it.

Integration is linked with the idea that a problem comes into counselling described in the client's best language for translating their experience. Systemic counselling invites us to consider the meaning behind the client's language, at times even word by word, and what the word-meanings convey of the client's social identity, family history, life stage, and cultural knowledge. Translating the client's experience into circular and relational concepts has the effect of the client reframing and re-experiencing their identity, family background, life situation, and culture. But systemic translations come with remarkable limits. They miss the depth of a person's experience. They ignore the reality of the problem inside the client's thoughts, feelings, and behaviours. And they cannot articulate the individual growth of a client.

The SIC model comes with the belief that it is beneficial to work on the relationships around the problem as well as the deeper experience of the client. Taking

DOI: 10.4324/9781003480808-11

a *systemic* breadth approach means seeing the broader interaction patterns that create ruptures in a person's wellbeing. The complementary *individualistic* depth approach means an orientation of probing into the distress, hidden feelings, and unconscious motivations that obscure the client's positive psychological outlook. Using Burnham's AMT model has allowed me to create systemic integrative counselling by moving those depth techniques into a systemic approach or theory.

Systems Theory

In this section we are going to meet a client named Alex. She describes herself as a kind and friendly person who wishes to do well by others. In counselling she is exploring an anxious hesitation at confronting people in her life, feeling unable to stand up for herself, resisting conflict at the expense of loosening her boundaries. Other people take advantage of her agreeable nature by making unfair demands. In the room she tears up paper while she talks about a colleague at work who expects her to tidy up his mess. As a systemic counsellor I consider ways to unpack the relationship dynamics between her and her colleague, asking circular questions:

"How do you respond when he expects you to tidy up his mess?"
"What does he do when you tidy up after him?"
"How does he show his expectation of you tidying up?"

The theory underpinning SIC is systems theory, which defines a system as a complicated set of things working together in a connected whole. For example, the work system is a complex set of managers, workers, administrators, policy makers, and customers, working together in a retail network. The school system is a complicated set of teachers, students, support workers, governors, and parents, working together in a connected educational network. A family system is a set of mums, dads, brothers, sisters, dogs, aunts, and so on, working together as a network of relatives. Each system is made up of members, and each member contributes to keeping the system stable.

Alex is invited to map out her work system using circular questions that link her actions with those of her colleague into patterns that create meanings. What meanings led Alex to an anxiety about standing up for herself? In systems theory, systems are divided into subsystems. A parent and child make up one subsystem of a family. Two siblings make up another. The behaviour of the subsystem is very intricate and is determined by at least three things. First there is how the members of the system bond or work together. Then there are the rules that govern how the members interact within the system. And finally, there are the ways the members of the system communicate between bonding and setting relationship boundaries. By questioning how Alex responds to her colleague's demands, she gains insight into the underlying rules of this subsystem and her influence on the overall relationship.

A system is kept stable around interaction patterns in ways that become stereotyped and predictable. For example, a colleague subsystem that has the rule "Alex is responsible for cleaning" will interact in a way that frequently confirms this rule, no matter how the interaction begins. The colleague may demand that Alex cleans up, despite having the same job role as her. And she accepts the demand. Or the colleague may clean the work area rather loudly and frustratedly, as perceived by Alex, and she complains to him, stepping in and taking over. Had we described an individual in the colleague pair, we would have missed the systemic nature of their behaviours. One colleague might be called rude or inattentive, the other might be called a complainer or a perfectionist. But together we see there is a pattern, and the pattern is governed by an implicit rule.

In systems theory, there are two main types of interaction pattern that characterise systems and subsystems. Complementary, where behaviours are different in nature but complement each other. And mutual, where behaviours grow or shrink together. Two people arguing is a mutual relationship and one person arguing while the other remains silent is complementary. In systems theory, the behaviour and experience of one individual is describable in terms of the interaction patterns they are involved in. For example, when Alex is annoyed with her colleague, she may ignore him. Let's imagine that the colleague ignores her back. This mutual escalation could fizzle out if one person decides to reciprocate and behave complementarily, such as by reaching out to break the silence. Or usually by the tidying up stacking to a point of breaking down Alex's resistance. If the colleague had responded differently, by badgering Alex, for example, by making demands of her, this complementary pattern could also have escalated. Again, if one person decides to reciprocate, to break the pattern, the escalation dissolves. Though sometimes at the expense of at least one person's mental health. Reciprocity is essential to prevent systems and relationships from running away under their own steam and breaking apart.

A profound finding developed out of this relational view: the intensity and character of a client's mental health problem is to do with interaction patterns plus the level of escalation in their relationships. Had either of the above patterns kept escalating, we'd expect a chronically frustrated Alex or a chronically withdrawn Alex. Seeing the client outside of the systemic context could misguide a counsellor. A second profound finding is that patterns occur in contexts, and this brings us to another founding principle of systems theory.

The set of rules that people live by is determined by their family history and their culture. And so, the colleague pair may have the rule "Alex is responsible for cleaning", but where does this come from?

We ask Alex about her family history and her cultural identity, and she begins to make connections to places where this rule was learned. In her case, she is an older sibling of two younger brothers in her single-parent family home. She has often felt positioned as a step-parent in her family, being asked to tidy up after them and look after them when her mother is not home. Equally, as a female, she has been trapped inside a cultural belief that females do more of the cleaning. Thus, the work system is part of Alex's re-enactment of cultural and family values that explain some aspects of her problem with her colleague. Now we can link conversations about the work colleague to conversations about Alex's family and wider cultural experience.

In systems theory, the context is a crucial part of the change process. When clients live by self-defeating rules or narratives, they experience psychological problems. Clients learn to see their systems differently, to redraw the contract, renegotiate the rules, and live in new and more hopeful points of view. Thus, systems theory is a collection of ideas that begins with the view that individual psychological problems develop from circular social interactions. How people interact is defined by a social context. Systemic counselling is about working on the way people interact as well as the meaning and understanding they bring to their ways of interacting.

But after speaking with Alex and gaining some understanding of parts of her reality, she continues to tear up the paper on the table. There appears to be a feeling beyond her awareness that systems thinking has not quite grasped. A feeling that this way of working has no language for. At this juncture, I would want to bring in some tools for exploring her inner experience. Perhaps my approach can be more open to the bodily sensations and behaviour in the room?

System-Centred Counselling

The first step that SIC makes is to integrate client-centred approaches with systemic approaches. A counsellor thinks about the concept of circularity in a way that aims to build interpersonal awareness with the client. Achieving this is possible with circular questions, which are questions that map out interaction patterns. For instance, a client who says they have been feeling upset in some context like their home environment would be invited to verbalise sequences involving the anxiety. When you show anxiety, how does your mother respond? If your mum gives you comfort immediately, what does your dad do? When your dad tells your mum to leave you alone, what do you think about his actions? These circular questions develop systemic insight with clients and unpack the rules and roles that govern mental health problems.

The limits of circular questioning are clear to a person-centred therapist. How do we centre on the client's experience? When will the counsellor consider going deeper into the client's distress?

A system-centred approach uses systems theory to describe client issues and borrows techniques from client-centred counselling to expand the client's awareness, develop empathy, and ensure the client experiences unconditional positive regard. The systemic counsellor, having mapped out the interaction patterns, at any moment of heightened emotion or use of rich words probes further into the client's experience. The use of open questions, probing questions, paraphrasing, restating, and summarising then pushes the systemic technique beyond its boundary into a more individualistic, humanistic frame. That is, returning to Alex and her position in her family, the system-centred counsellor asks questions like "what emotion do you feel when your colleague or mother expects you to clean the mess?" (circular question), "how are you experiencing that emotion now?" (open question), "you say it's frustrating, what is frustrating about it?" (probing question), "it seems your colleague or mother expecting you to tidy up other people's mess is frustrating for you because you feel devalued and invalidated" (summarising statement).

System-centred counselling requires an ability to map the system, unpack the context for the interactions, and dive into the experiential world of the client as they experience things from within the system. Insofar as we have combined systemic counselling with person-centred counselling, adding in person-centred techniques to a systemic perspective, we have resolved the issue of having no tools for probing into the client's experience. But sometimes even those two attempts to connect with clients' experiences fall flat, and the client rejects the approach or shuts down, particularly when opening painful feelings. Counsellors are often baffled as to why a careful circular question or probing statement is rejected by the client, and sometimes the client provokes good therapists into feeling hopeless or unstable. Alex may become frustrated with us, and we respond with a complementary pattern by attempting to show more empathy or curiosity, thus increasing her withdrawing or frustrating behaviour. A psychodynamic counsellor has tools on offer to consider this situation, and the SIC approach encourages bringing in these tools to the therapeutic relationship.

Psychosystemic Counselling

The psychodynamic idea that childhood experiences fuse into an unconscious template and set of responses for meeting and communicating needs of a biological, sociological, and psychological nature can also can be integrated with systems theory. The psychosystemic counsellor notices interaction patterns for how clients respond to care, authority figures, and relationships in general and points out these patterns in the hope of creating insight with the client. After the counselling has made some progress in mapping out the system around the problem, using circular questions, the present behaviour of the client can be reflected on in terms of what the behaviour reveals about the underlying structures of the client's experience.

Systems theory and psychodynamic theory are different in description, but they can work together. For instance, when Alex responds to a careful question with frustration, and to empathy with agitation, and to openness with being closed off, we might do well to unpack this repeated pattern in the room. A psychodynamic perspective would name this as transference and guess at the fact that the client is showing defence mechanisms due to unresolved anger towards caregivers. At the unconscious level, the client is re-creating negative experiences of care. Systemically, the description simply moves from the unconscious template to the non-conscious interaction pattern. That is, the client converts the counsellor into being a frustrated caregiver by using complementary escalations. The better the counsellor, the more shutdown the client.

In working with transference and countertransference, the SIC model uses relational reflexivity. As well as offering interpretations as a therapeutic tool, as the psychodynamic counsellor might, relational reflexivity highlights the observation, interpretable as transference, and enquires about the impact, meaning, and desires of the client. That is, relational reflexivity takes feedback from the client's shutting down and converts it into a circular intervention. "When I did that just now, how was that for you?", "What sort of questions would be most useful today?", "I am unsure if we are on the right track; how would you like the counselling to move forward from here?". These questions invite reflection on the relationship between client and counsellor and reveal many of the same unconscious processes. Clients will tell the counsellor they were being rude, too direct, or unhelpful. Provided the counsellor can hear feedback in the context of childhood and earlier relationships, it can detangle the countertransference and help clients work on their relationship to help: "is this frustration and disappointment a common feeling you get when you reach out for help or is it just here in this moment?".

The concept of relational reflexivity is congruent with systemic counselling. It means to enquire about the meaning and experience a person is having or imagines having in counselling. It is important to remind ourselves of the guiding principles, that SIC is a systemic-contextual approach using techniques from counselling modalities. To avoid being inconsistent in how therapy works, as in to avoid being a different therapist each week with the client, we encourage a systemic outlook as the overriding theme of SIC techniques. Thus, stepping into the unconscious process or the client's experience is seen as probing into one component of the relationship system. We are not breaking with the systemic perspective, simply taking a microscope to part of the system to reveal some important features with the client.

A psychodynamic approach would make connections between current relationship experiences and previous relationships. This too is congruent with SIC. For instance, the activity called Malan's Triangle connects the response to the counsellor and a current or historic relationship. "Is your frustration with seeking my help similar to when you seek help from your manager?", "Is the way you expect your manager to be annoyed with you when you state your needs similar to how you felt your mother was annoyed at you when you needed help?". I call this a psychosystemic approach because it views the psychological disposition, such as a hesitant relationship with care, in terms of the system, and it works on the deeper issues and the relational issues together. Using concepts like the id or instinctive impulses, the ego or conscious reality, and the superego or unconscious set of internalised rules can further assist clients in interpreting their reality while remaining curious about the relationship patterns that govern the unconscious mind. Psychodynamic therapy might call the structure of the mind, the id, ego, and superego, a theoretical account of personality, and SIC suggests seeing them as techniques, ways of intervening with clients to contribute to positive change.

Contextual Behaviour Therapy

The rise of cognitive-behavioural therapy (CBT) has cast a shadow on much of the other counselling modalities within health services. And this is for a good reason.

Not because it is superior, although some people do make this claim, but because CBT is measurable and practical in a way that no other counselling modality can rival. This is because the concepts in CBT are easy to see. They are behaviours. We can only measure the unconscious by interpreting behaviour. We can only measure psychological growth by interpreting behaviour. CBT takes away the need for interpretation and as such is more easily integrated into the science of counselling compared with other models.

CBT is an intra-systemic modality. It works on the cognitive system, the circularity of the thought, feeling, behaviour cycles. As well as being easy to study, this also makes it a good candidate for integrating with systems theory. In fact, one could argue that cognitive-behavioural cycles are microsystems of the individual. The individual is a biological system, including a cognitive system, of a family, and a family is a subsystem of a community. Moving this on, following Bronfenbrenner's ecological systems theory, we notice that the community is part of a wider region and an even wider national culture. From the negative intrusive thought all the way to the cultural values of success, attractiveness, and intelligence, there is an interconnected thread.

This is why SIC says that behaviour happens in a context. A thought is a behaviour. An emotion is shown behaviourally. A behaviour is, of course, a behaviour. Taking a presenting problem like an inability to stand up for oneself, we see that anxious behaviours happen only within certain contexts. For instance, a work context that places value on women being cleaners and tidiers but not decision makers. Alex said that she did not have the same anxiety with her boyfriend; in fact he described her as bossy and strong, someone who can absolutely stand up for herself.

Integrating CBT with systems theory means processing a client's cognitive cycles in relation to their social context and interaction patterns. The Circular Hot Cross Bun is an activity that illustrates the ingenuity of combining cognitive theory with systems theory. In this therapeutic activity, the client visualises the presenting problem in a specific time and place. Let's move away from Alex for now, and work with a different problem. For example, "low mood" while a client is out at a family party.

In this activity, the client draws the important people on an A4 page. Now the traditional cognitive-behaviour intervention, the hot cross bun model, is drawn with the client (see Figure 10.1). They write down their thoughts. Something like "I am not sociable, everyone here is going to think I am being rude". Their feelings, "I am nervous and a bit on edge". Their behaviour, "I sit on my own and don't talk much". So far, we are helping the client to use psychoeducation, to learn about their cognitions in a way that develops them psychologically. And this is a CBT modality that the SIC uses as an intervention. Reminding ourselves that SIC translates integrative counselling tools into a systemically informed approach.

To cast the activity into a systemic frame, we ask the client to consider the social world around him. What do you imagine are the other people's cognitive cycles? The client draws or explains them. And we support the client, using

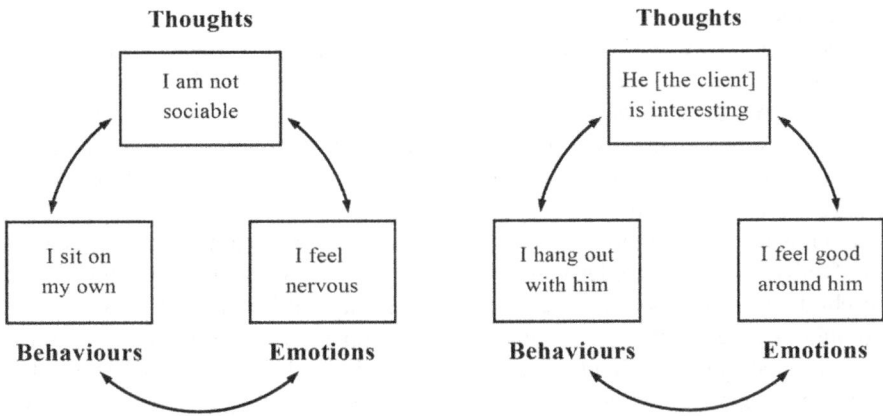

Figure 10.1 Relational Hot Cross Bun Example

circular questions, to consider how his intrusive thinking and avoidant behaviour are impacted by the context around him. Then, following the CBT pathway, we challenge the thoughts or put them on trial, unpack them with questions, or consider trialling some behaviour experiments. Here we ask the client to consider how different thoughts and different behaviours might help construct new social realities. And this is the crux of the contextual behavioural approach. We ask, "If you thought that your cousin would find your story about work interesting, how might this affect your feeling about being in the party?", "When you think of yourself as being rude, how do other people feel around you?". These *circular* questions situate a person and their cognitive-behavioural cycles back into a relational frame.

The SIC model places emphasis on the counselling technique being used or understood in a circular way. This is why person-centred questions are made circular, psychodynamic interpretations are made relational, and CBT activities are used to highlight patterns. But SIC also draws on the long history of systemic therapy, particularly around family therapy and narrative therapy.

Family Counselling

A problem such as low mood enters the relationship system via the family structure. This is because families are organised into patterns of relating and responding to people depending on their position within the family. Two family members who bond together are said to be in an alliance. A supportive aunt or a caring uncle. A safe haven at grandma's house, or a parent who fights your corner. But alliances are generally part of wider family structures and can be veiled coalitions, relationships that look nice from within the relationship but have some negative effects outside of it.

The most basic structure of a family is a two-person subsystem. Watch how a mother responds when a father enters the room. Or how a father responds when a son enters the room. In these micro-moments, people show their true relational colours. Does the mother invite or dismiss the father's company? Does the father mock or celebrate his son's presence? And how does the son respond to the father? Interaction patterns between two people are often part of a three-person triangle. This means that two people can gang up into a coalition against one person, where their alliance serves the function of going against another person in the family. For instance, let's imagine a mother with a low tolerance for distress in children. When looking after her infant child, who becomes distressed about an unknown cause, possibly food, possibly sickness, she begins to get frustrated and stressed, perhaps shouting, or becoming distant from the child. The father, in noticing this, addresses the mother's behaviour by asking her to connect more with the child's distress or to speak more calmly. The mother responds to the father with an escalation in stress and a lower tolerance for distress. He escalates too, becoming more critical and removing the child from her care. The child and their father form a coalition against the mother, and this is a triangulated system (Figure 10.2).

The situation can become triangulated if every time the child shows distress, including when the child is now a 30-year-old adult, the mother becomes stressed and the father criticises her, taking back the caring role. The father and son may even talk about how stressful the mother is and be perplexed as to why she cannot keep calm. The triangulation is now a pattern that involves creating a stressed mother, a distressed or anxious son, and a frustrated father. In family counselling, we support the family or individual client to map out their interaction patterns by using a genogram or by unpacking interactions through circular questions.

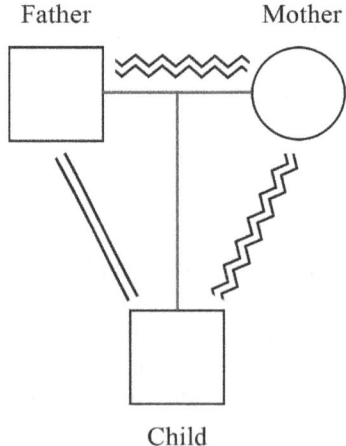

Figure 10.2 Triangulation

Usually, the client struggles with this circular way of thinking. The SIC model encourages a spontaneous movement through person-centred, psychodynamic, and CBT ideas, because this encourages the client to develop relational thinking while validating and accepting other ways of perceiving things. For example, I met a client who formed a coalition with their mother against their father. I asked a circular question of the kind, "when your father gets angry at your mother, how do you respond?". The client said that they would comfort their mother, usually when things have cooled down, by providing hugs and not speaking with dad for a while. An unforeseen effect of the question was to raise the client's suspicion that I was being too empathic with dad, indirectly criticising the mother-daughter relationship. And she may well have a point there!

SIC gives the systemic counsellor permission to consider the transference in the room, whereby I was being experienced with the same anxiety as when speaking with her father, and my maleness was tainting my genuine intention to care. Here we could have explored that. Or the countertransference in the room; perhaps my relationship with my father or my relationship as a father was colouring how I evaluated the mother-daughter bond? I could have unpacked the thought-feeling-behaviour cycles and found some way forward with this. Instead, I chose a person-centred route, asking how it was when I empathised with dad. She said she felt misunderstood and as though her worry for her mother was being seen as overdramatic.

Taking the person-centred route, I probed into the word "overdramatic", and the client became aware of how her father had called her overdramatic many times and it was his common word for describing her mother. We unpacked, in a client-led way, the experience of being labelled overdramatic, raising my empathy, moving to a position of unconditional positive regard. I really felt for her and wanted to accept her experience. The result was the client being free from the grip of the "overdramatic" description in our therapeutic relationship, because in the process of caring about the description I was not replicating a critical patriarch. An important effect of this was that the client was more interested in and receptive to the circular questions, naming times where she does feel her relationship with her mother pushes her father away, and times where she gives comfort to her mother when she feels her mother is in the wrong. SIC responds to the restraints in systems thinking, essentially in the neutrality of the counsellor, by showing how some clients can feel misunderstood or criticised when asked about their role in the relationship. Switching to a person-centred set of skills is one of a variety of ways to keep family counselling going while attending to experiences along the way.

Family counselling keeps a focus on the familial aspects of the presenting problem. The counsellor works on the family structure through alliances, coalitions, subsystems, interaction patterns, and hierarchy. And they map out how the structure changes with time. The predictable changes are events like coupling, marriage, birth of children, becoming a parent, school, adulthood, and death. These are life cycles that create a need for families to change their structure. Either because someone moves out of the home or dies, and the interactions between the remaining family members change, new hierarchies and alliances form, or because someone moves in, perhaps through marriage or birth, and this new person shakes up the system.

Language, Communication, and Action

One of the key ideas in family counselling is family scripts. It rests on the theory that family members are a communication system and a language system. Communication theory is broken down into three parts. Part 1 is the technical level for how accurately things are transmitted from one location to another. Part 2 is the semantic level for how accurately the meaning of the things or symbols is conveyed. Part 3 is the effectiveness level for how effectively the received meaning affects the behaviour of the receiver of the signal. Language is the main form of communication within families although behaviour and body language also constitute a fair amount of communication.

Family scripts combines language and communication theory into an explanation for why family members fall into predictable interaction sequences. When people communicate, they become more and more efficient, such that people who know one another can simply raise an eyebrow or let out a short puff of air to convey a complex message. In a sense, people rehearse communication over and over again until they establish a routine that cuts the transfer of meaning down to the essentials. For instance, a new partner who wants to express feelings might, in the beginning, take a while to explain the feeling and the context for the feeling, with some apology and tangential remarks. Over time, the feeling, whether it be anxiety or excitement, will be expressed quickly through the use of shared symbols like ignoring a text message for ten minutes or sitting by the window when their partner arrives. In systems theory, this is called redundancy where the essential parts of the intended message are communicated, and the rest become unnecessary or redundant. When there is redundancy in the system, people begin to act from stereotyped emotions, positions, and roles. That is, in a family context a person begins to live as though they are acting out a script. And each time they behave like themselves, they are rehearsing the same script over and over.

The variety of scripts is endless, whether they be parental scripts, partnership scripts, scripts about gender roles or confidence levels, scripts about moral positions and individual rights, but family scripts theory categorises them into three main types. First, there are scripts that are repeated from generation to generation or from society to individual, and these are called replicative scripts. Scripts that repeat the dialogue and actions from other contexts. Second, there are scripts that correct and challenge family and social scripts, and these are called corrective scripts. These are usually due to a bad or oppressive experience for having lived within the parameters of an earlier script, such as correcting a negative parenting experience. The final type of script is called improvised, where a person has the freedom and autonomy to create their own unique script within a given situation.

To unpack family scripts, SIC draws from integrative counselling techniques. Systemically, the counsellor might think about how scripts position clients into narratives, stories, or roles. And how these stories or roles generate certain inter-personal patterns. Humanistically, the counsellor unpacks the family script with a depth lens, digging beneath the experience. For instance, they may draw the ice-berg model with the client, in which the script is written into the tip of an ice-berg and the client lists and draws the experiences, feelings, worries, connections, memories, under the surface.

Being congruent with a systemic approach, SIC is system focused, being ori-ented towards using techniques and concepts relationally. Thus, when thinking about family counselling, a SIC approach encourages the counsellor to work with the systemic components of a family. These are communication, flexibility, and rules or boundaries. What are your scripts around being a parent? How does this influence the way you set rules as a parent? In what ways do you communicate? Thus, SIC is about stepping into techniques from counselling modalities while holding in mind the system.

Action and Embodiment Counselling

The nature of SIC is an evolving set of techniques within a systemic approach. It is never finished. In its current iteration, the last part of an SIC approach is action-embodiment counselling. Humanistic and person-centred approaches have probed into the experience of the client but, so far, we have not used action as a way of embodying and processing, bodily, the client's experiences and meaning systems. We have explored the social reality, the cognitive reality, the behavioural reality, the unconscious needs and interpretations, but have not yet harnessed the bodily reality of the client or allowed the body to tell its story.

Action techniques are those interventions that use the body or objects to act out, symbolise, represent, dramatise, and visualise a client's experience or relationship system. The client embodies their world of experience via dramatic techniques. For instance, in sculpting, a client uses themself and their family members, or some symbolic substitute for family members, to sculpt the family relationships as they see and experience them. People may be distant or close. They may be angry or sad. Some people are represented as higher or lower in stature and seating position. Family splits, coalitions, and histories of abuse are shown through posture and barricades placed between people. This systemic technique attends to the visceral embodied reality of the client. And, frequently in counselling, actions speak louder than words.

Systemic techniques can be turned into action techniques if used in dramatic and creative ways. For instance, instead of asking a circular question, which aims to map out interaction patterns within the relationship system, the client can enact the interaction live in the therapy room with a real or imaged member of the relation-ship. This technique, which is called enactment, allows the client to relive ways of relating to others while the counsellor gains information about the types of scripts, life cycles, thoughts, feelings, coalitions, and interaction sequences which are con-tributing to the presenting problem. If the client is an individual and not a couple or a family then they can use the empty chair method, from gestalt therapy, to hold the conversation as they remember and imagine it. Doing so, the SIC counsellor has permission to notice the phenomenology of hand gestures, voice tones, and body language, and to invite the client to express and reflect on these aspects of their relationships. The counsellor may also, as with gestalt therapy, have the client take different symbols or projections from their drama to work on. For instance, if a client plays out an interaction with a sibling in which they are displaying low self-worth, the counsellor might have the client put "low self-worth" in the opposite chair and support an interaction. Focusing on the present moment is an important aspect of SIC that fits with a systemic model if the relationship system is the primary way of understanding the therapy process.

Action techniques provide the space for the client to show meaning and experience through bodily expression, drama, and use of space. Asking the client to scale out of 10 how anxious they are feeling brings forward one aspect of their reality; asking them to view the room as a scale, with 1 at one side of the room and 10 at another side, encourages them to represent spatially, to embody the scale and express its deeper meaning. In SIC we are encouraging an openness to the multiplicity of meanings that clients bring into the counselling room, suggesting that all modalities create therapeutic possibilities for counsellors to draw on.

Conclusion

Systemic Integrative Counselling views counselling modalities as tools and techniques to use in circular and systemic ways. The starting point with the SIC approach is based on the decision the counsellor makes about the most suitable fit with the client. In SIC, the counsellor may start with a systemic approach and probe into a CBT cycle or an unconscious process, or with a phenomenological enquiry and end with a question about meaning and purpose. Techniques are integrated into a bigger picture of counselling under the banner of systemic integrative counselling. As a SIC counsellor, it has felt valuable to give myself permission to step in and out of different counselling models. I have felt restricted by my favourite ideas and empowered by the counselling ideas that clash most with my outlook. It is my view that clients deserve to have experienced counsellors who are specialised in their way of working. Of course! But I hope this book has demonstrated that whatever your guiding counselling philosophy is, you can borrow ideas from any modality to work on different aspects of the bigger picture, providing you take the technique and use it within your counselling theory. SIC is one of a variety of expressions of integrative counselling that values the wide lens of relationships, family, and society, as well as the zoom lens of experience, unconscious process, action, and embodiment.

Counselling is as much an art as it is a science. We will never have a complete theory of counselling and our practices will continue to grow and develop in endless directions. I am hopeful the model in this book inspires counsellors to think beyond the limits of the approaches they have learned and to create new and meaningful ways to bring more hope and wellbeing to the lives of their clients. In ending this book, I hope counsellors and therapists have enriched their practice, made sense out of how to combine different techniques into a meaningful approach, and have the permission to experiment with their unique counselling and psychotherapy approaches.

References

Anderson, H., & Goolishian, H. (1992). The client is the expert: A not-knowing approach to therapy. In S. McNamee & K. J. Gergen (Eds.), *Therapy as social construction* (pp. 25–39). London: Sage Publications, Inc.

Anderson, T. (1995). *Reflecting processes; Acts of informing and forming. You can borrow my eyes but you must not take them away from me!* New York: The Guilford Press.

Austin, J. L. (1962). *How to do things with words*. Oxford: Clarendon.

Bachler, E., Frühmann, A., Bachler, H., Aas, B., Strunk, G., & Nickel, M. (2016). Differential effects of the working alliance in family therapeutic home-based treatment of multi-problem families. *Journal of Family Therapy, 38*, 120–148. doi:10.1111/1467-6427.12063.

Bateson, G. (1972). *Steps to an ecology of mind*. San Francisco: Chandler.

Bateson, G. (1980). *Mind and nature. A necessary unity*. New York: Bantam Books.

Baucom, D. H., Belus, J. M., Adelman, C. B., Fischer, M. S., & Paprocki, C. (2014), Couple-based interventions for psychopathology: A renewed direction for the field. *Family Process, 53*, 445–461. doi:10.1111/famp.12075.

Beck, A. T. (1993). Cognitive therapy: Past, present, and future. *Journal of Consulting and Clinical Psychology, 61*(2), 194–198. doi:10.1037/0022-006X.61.2.194.

Bertalanffy, L. von. (1968). *General system theory: Foundation, development, application.* New York: George Braziller.

Boroditsky, L., Schmidt, L., & Phillips, W. (2003). Sex, syntax, and semantics. In D. Gentner & S. Goldin-Meadow (Eds.), *Language in mind: Advances in the study of language and cognition* (pp. 61–79). Cambridge, MA: MIT Press.

Bowen, M. (1985). *Family therapy in clinical practice*. Lanham, MD: Rowman and Littlefield.

Bronfenbrenner, U. (1979). *The ecology of human development: Experiments by nature and design*. Cambridge, MA: Harvard University Press.

Burnham, J. (1986). *Family therapy*. London: Routledge.

Burnham, J. (1992). Approach – method – technique: Making distinctions and creating connections. *Human Systems: The Journal of Systemic Consultation & Management, 3*, 3–26.

Burnham, J. (2000). Internalized other interviewing: Evaluating and enhancing empathy. *Clinical Psychology Forum, 140*, 16–20.

Burnham, J. (2005). *Relational reflexivity: A tool for socially constructing therapeutic relationships*. London: Karnac Books.

Burnham, J. (2012). Developments in social GRRRAAACCEEESSS: Visible – invisible and voiced – Unvoiced. In I.-B. Krause (Ed.), *Mutual perspectives: Culture and reflexivity in contemporary systemic psychotherapy* (pp. 139–160). London: Karnac.

Burr, V. (2015). *Social constructionism* (3rd ed.). London: Routledge.

Byng-Hall, J. (1985). The family script: A useful bridge between theory and practice. *Journal of Family Therapy*, 7(3), 301–305.

Carter, B., & McGoldrick, M. (Eds.). (1988). *The changing family life cycle: A framework for family therapy* (2nd ed.). New York: Gardner Press.

Carr, A. (2014). The evidence-base for family therapy and systemic interventions for child focused problems. *Journal of Family Therapy*, 36, 107–157.

Carr, A. (2014). The evidence-base for couple therapy, family therapy and systemic interventions for adult-focused problems. *Journal of Family Therapy*, 36, 158–194.

Carr, A., Pinquart, M., & Haun, M. W. (2020). Research-informed practice of systemic therapy. In M. Ochs, M. Borcsa, & J. Schweitzer (Eds.), *Systemic research in individual, couple and family therapy and counseling* (pp. 319–347). Cham: Springer.

Cecchin, G. (1987). Hypothesizing, circularity and neutrality revisited. An invitation to curiosity. *Family Process*, 24(1), 15–25.

Chomsky, N. (2006). *Language and mind* (3rd ed.). Cambridge University Press. doi:10.1017/CBO9780511791222.

Cooper, M (2010). *Essential research findings in counselling and psychotherapy: The facts are friendly*. London: Sage Publications Ltd.

Elliott, R., Greenberg, L., & Lietaer, G. (2004). Research on experiential psychotherapies. In M. Lambert (Ed.), *Bergin and Garfield's handbook of psychotherapy and behaviour change* (5th ed., pp. 493–539). New York: Wiley.

de Maat, S., de Jonghe, F., Schoevers, R., & Dekker, J. (2009). The effectiveness of long-term psychoanalytic therapy: A systematic review of empirical studies. *Harvard Review of Psychiatry*, 17, 1–23. doi:10.1080/16073220902742476.

Durkheim, É. (1984). *The division of labour in society* (2nd ed.). New York: Macmillan.

Faris, A., & Ooijen, E. Van. (2012). *Integrative counselling and psychotherapy: A textbook*. London: Routledge.

Fordham, B., Sugavanam, T., Edwards, K., Stallard, P., Howard, R., Das Nair, R., … Lamb, S. (2021). The evidence for cognitive behavioural therapy in any condition, population or context: A meta-review of systematic reviews and panoramic meta-analysis. *Psychological Medicine*, 51(1), 21–29. doi:10.1017/S0033291720005292.

Foucault, M. (1965). *Madness and civilization: A history of insanity in the age of reason*. New York: Pantheon Books.

Fox, K. (2004). *Watching the English, the hidden rules of English behaviour*. London: Hodder and Stoughton.

Freud, S. (1977). An outline of psychoanalysis. In J. Strachey (Ed.), *The standard edition of the complete psychological works of Sigmund Freud* (Vol. 23, pp. 139–207). London: Hogarth Press.

Greenberger, D., & Padesky, C. (1995). *Mind over mood: Changing how you feel by changing the way you think*. New York: Guilford.

Gurman, A. S., & Burton, M. (2014). Individual therapy for couple problems: Perspectives and pitfalls. *Journal of Marital and Family Therapy*, 38, 470–483. doi:10.1111/jmft.12061.

Haley, J., & Richeport-Haley, M. (2003). *The art of strategic therapy*. New York: Routledge.

Hardy, K. V., & Laszloffy, T. A. (1995). The cultural genogram: Key to training culturally competent family therapists. *The Journal of Marital & Family Therapy, 21*(3), 227–237.

Hare-Mustin, R. T. (1994). Discourses in the mirrored room: A postmodern analysis of therapy. *Family Process, 33*, 19–35. doi:10.1111/j.1545-5300.1994.00019.x.

Harré, R., & Van Langenhove, L. (Eds.). (1999). *Positioning theory.* Oxford: Blackwell.

Hornsby, D. (2014). *Linguistics, a complete introduction.* London: Hodder and Stoughton.

Husserl, E. (1989). *Ideas pertaining to a pure phenomenology and to a phenomenological philosophy.* Boston: Springer.

Kierkegaard, S. (1959). *Either/or.* New York: Doubleday.

King, M., Sibbald, B., Ward, E., Bower, P., Lloyd, M., Gabbey, M., et al. (2000). Randomised control trials of non-directive counselling, cognitive-behaviour therapy and usual general practitioner care in the management of depression as well as mixed anxiety and depression in primary care. *Health Technology Assessment, 19*(1), 1–83.

Koganei, K., Asaoka, Y., Nishimatsu, Y., & Kito, S. (2021), Women's psychological experiences in a narrative therapy-based group: An analysis of participants' writings and beck depression inventory–second edition. *Japanese Psychological Research, 63*, 466–475. doi:10.1111/jpr.12326.

Konorski, J. (1967). *Integrative activity of the brain.* Chicago: University of Chicago Press.

Lang, P., & McAdam, E. (1997). Narrative-ating: Future dreams in present living, jottings on an honouring theme. *Human Systems: The Journal of Systemic Consultation and Management, 8*(1), 3–12.

Lang, P., & McAdam, E. (2009). *Appreciative work in schools.* West Sussex: Kingsham Press.

Lapworth, P., & Sills, C. (2009). *Integration in counselling psychotherapy: Developing a personal approach.* London: Sage.

Leichsenring, F., & Rabung, S. (2008). Effectiveness of long-term psychodynamic psychotherapy: A meta-analysis. *Journal of the American Medical Association, 300*, 1551–1565.

Lewin, K. (2008). *Resolving social conflicts and field theory in social science.* Washington, DC: American Psychological Association.

Lopes, R. T., Gonçalves, M. M., Machado, P., Sinai, D., Bento, T., & Salgado, J. (2014, November). Narrative therapy vs. Cognitive-behavioral therapy for moderate depression: Empirical evidence from a controlled clinical trial. *Psychotherapy Research, 24*(6), 662–674.

Luhmann, N. (2013). *Introduction to systems theory.* Cambridge: Polity Press.

Malan, D. (1995). *Individual psychotherapy and the science of psychodynamics.* Oxford: Butterworth-Heinemann.

Meadows, D. (2009). *Thinking in systems.* Vermont: Chelsea Green Publishing.

Milner, V., McIntosh, H., Colvert, E., & Happé, F. (2019). A qualitative exploration of the female experience of Autism Spectrum Disorder (ASD). *Journal of Autism and Developmental Disorders, 49*(6), 2389–2402. doi:10.1007/s10803-019-03906-4.

Minuchin, S. (2012). *Families and Family Therapy* (2nd ed.). London: Routledge. doi:10.4324/9780203111673.

Minuchin, S., & Nichols, M. P. (1993). *Family healing tales of hope and renewal from family therapy.* New York: Free Press.

Moodley, R., Sutherland, P., & Oulanova, O. (2008). Traditional healing, the body and mind in psychotherapy. *Counseling Psychology Quarterly*, *21*(2), 153–165. doi:10.1080/09515070802066870.

Moreno, J. L. (1946). *Psychodrama* (1st vols.). Beacon House. doi:10.1037/11506-000.

Moreno, J. L. (1994). *Psychodrama since moreno* (M. Karp & M. Watson, Eds.). London: Routledge.

Murphy, R. (2022). How children make sense of their permanent exclusion: A thematic analysis from semi-structured interviews. *Emotional and Behavioural Difficulties*, *27*(1), 43–57. doi:10.1080/13632752.2021.2012962.

Nichols, M. P., & Fellenberg, S. (2000). The effective use of enactments in family therapy: A discovery-oriented process study. *Journal of Marital and Family Therapy*, *26*, 143–152.

Olson, D. H. (1993). Circumplex model of marital and family systems: Assessing family functioning. In F. Walsh (Ed.), *Normal family processes* (pp. 104–137). The Guilford Press.

Papp, P., Scheinkman, M., & Malpas, J. (2013). Breaking the mold: Sculpting impasses in couples' therapy. *Family Process*, *52*, 33–45.

Parsons, T. (1951). *The social system*. Glenco, IL: Free Press.

Parsons, T. (1978). *Action theory and the human condition*. New York: Free Press.

Partridge, K. (2007). The positioning compass: A tool to facilitate reflexive positioning. *Human Systems: The Journal of Systemic Consultation and Management*, *18*, 96–111.

Pavlov, I. P. (1927). *Conditioned reflexes: An investigation of the physiological activity of the cerebral cortex*. Oxford: Oxford University Press.

Pearce, B. (2007). *Making social worlds: A communication perspective*. Malden, MA: Blackwell Publishers.

Perls, F. (1969). *Ego, hunger, and aggression; The beginning of gestalt therapy*. New York: Random House.

Perls, F., Hefferline, R., & Goodman, P. (1951). *Gestalt therapy: Excitement and growth in the human personality*. New York: Dell.

Rogers, C. (2020). *Client-centred therapy* (70th ed.). London: Robinson.

Rosen, K. H., Lechtenberg, M. M., & Stith, S. M. (2015). Strategic family therapy. In J. L. Wetchler & L. L. Hecker (Eds.), *An introduction to marriage and family therapy* (pp. 155–181). New York: Routledge.

Russell, W., Breunlin, D., & Sahebi, B. (2022). *Integrative systemic therapy*. London: Routledge.

Selvini, M.P., Boscolo, L., Cecchin, G., & Prata, G. (1980). Hypothesizing – circularity – neutrality: Three guidelines for the conductor of the session. *Family Process*, *19*(3), 12. doi:10.1111/j.1545-5300.1980.00003.x.

Shannon, C., & Weaver, W. (1998). *The mathematical theory of communication*. Oxford: Marston.

Skinner, B. F. (1988). *About behaviourism*. New York: Random House.

Staples, J., Atti, J., & Gordon, J. (2011). Mind-body skills groups for posttraumatic stress disorder and depression symptoms in Palestinian children and adolescents in Gaza. *International Journal of Stress Management*, *18*(2), 246–262. doi:10.1037/a0024015.

Starr, A. (1977). *Rehearsal for living: Psychodrama*. Chicago: Nelson Hall.

Stoddard, G. J. (2010). Outcome evaluation of the veterans affairs salt lake city integrative health clinic for chronic pain and stress-related depression, anxiety, and post-traumatic stress disorder. *Journal of Alternative & Complementary Medicine*, *16*(8), 823–835.

Stratton, P. (2016). *The evidence base of family therapy and systemic practice*. Warrington: Association of Family Therapy.

Tomm, K. M. (1987). Interventive interviewing: Part II. Reflexive questioning as a means to enable self-healing. *Family Process, 26*, 153–183. doi:10.1111/j.1545-5300.1987.00167.

Tomm, K. M. (1991). Beginnings of a "HIPs and PIPs" approach to psychiatric assessment. *The Calgary Participator, 1*(2), 21–24.

Truss, L. (2007). *Eats, shoots, and leaves*. London: Harper Collins.

Vromans, L. P., & Schweitzer, R. D. (2011). Narrative therapy for adults with major depressive disorder: Improved symptom and interpersonal outcomes. *Psychotherapy Research, 21*(1), 4–15. doi: 10.1080/10503301003591792.

Watzlawick, P., Weakland, J. W., & Fisch, R. (1974). *Change*. New York: W.W. Norton & Company.

Westen, D., Novotny, C. A., & Thompson-Brener, H. (2004). The empirical status of the empirically supported psychotherapies: Assumptions, findings and reporting in controlled clinical trials. *Psychological Bulletin, 130*(4), 631–633.

Wiener, N. (1948). *Cybernetics; or control and communication in the animal and the machine*. London: Wiley.

Williams, M., Teasdale, J., Segal, Z., & Kabat-Zinn, J. (2007). *The mindful way through depression: Freeing yourself from chronic unhappiness*. New York: The Guilford Press.

Wittgenstein, L. (1953). *Philosophical investigations*. Oxford: Blackwell.

Index

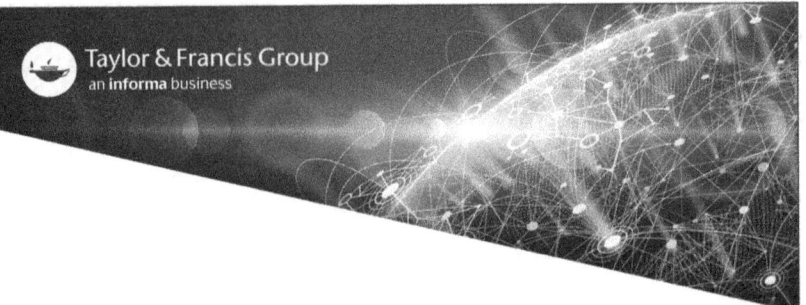
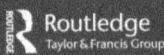
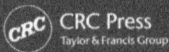